VETERINARY DENTISTRY
for the Technician & Office Staff

VETERINARY DENTISTRY
for the Technician & Office Staff

STEVEN E. HOLMSTROM, DVM

Diplomate, American Veterinary Dental College
San Carlos, California

SAUNDERS
An Imprint of Elsevier

SAUNDERS
An Imprint of Elsevier

The Curtis Center
Independence Square West
Philadelphia, Pennsylvania 19106

Library of Congress Cataloging–in–Publication Data

Holmstrom, Steven E.
    Veterinary dentistry for the technician & office staff / Steven E.
Holmstrom.
        p.   cm.
    Includes bibliographical references (p.   ) and index.
    ISBN 0-7216-8187-5
    1. Veterinary dentistry.   I. Title.
SF867.H76   1999
636.089′76—dc21   99-39640
                                                                        CIP

VETERINARY DENTISTRY
FOR THE TECHNICIAN AND OFFICE STAFF   ISBN 0-7216-8187-5

Printed in the United States of America

Last digit is the print number: 9 8 7 6 5 4

Contributors

LAURIE A. HOLMSTROM
Registered Dental Hygienist
Neubauer, Stolpa, and Pelzar Clinical Practice
San Carlos, California

CHARLES J. MCGRATH, DVM
Diplomate, American College of Veterinary Anesthesiologists
Professor
Virginia Tech, Virginia-Maryland Regional College of Veterinary Medicine
Department of Small Animal Clinical Sciences
Blacksburg, Virginia

MEGHAN T. RICHEY, DVM, MS
Diplomate, American College of Veterinary Anesthesiologists
Assistant Professor
Oklahoma State University
College of Veterinary Clinical Sciences
Stillwater, Oklahoma

ROBERT BRUCE WIGGS, BS, DVM
Diplomate, American Veterinary Dental College
Adjunct Associate Professor
Department of Biomedical Sciences
Baylor College of Dentistry, Texas A&M University Systems
Dallas, Texas

Owner
Dallas Dental Service Animal Clinic
12600 Coit Road
Dallas, Texas 75251

President, American Veterinary Dental College

Preface

As the practice of veterinary dentistry continues to evolve, more responsibilities will be delegated to veterinary office staff. The contributions of technicians are vital to the expansion of services and the completion of many dental-related tasks. One can find a great deal of satisfaction in being responsible for improving the dental department, including increasing the related productivity of the laboratory, anesthesia, radiology, dentistry, hospitalization, pharmacy, and retail departments. Dentistry is only one of the duties of today's well-trained technician, and it is a discipline that technicians can master, benefiting not only themselves but also their practice and its patients.

Veterinary Dentistry for the Technician and Office Staff was written to meet the needs of the registered veterinary technician and the entire office staff in the field of veterinary dentistry. It is intended to be comprehensive, bringing the student or already working technician, assistant, or receptionist from relatively little knowledge in veterinary dentistry to a practical, working knowledge. The chapters have been organized to help the reader progress from basic to more complex information. New terms and phrases are defined in brackets throughout the text rather than in a glossary that must be flipped back and forth to read. Tables emphasize essential information and present it to the reader in a concise, well-organized format. Photos and line drawings illustrate important concepts. One illustration shows the oral structures in a photograph with an overlaying drawing to demonstrate its key components. A unique and thus far unpublished dental chart allows successive visits to be documented on one chart rather than on separate charts or labels. Worksheets at the end of each chapter help the reader retain key information and improve skill competency.

This text was developed after having taught registered veterinary technicians and veterinary technician students for more than 10 years at Foothill College in Los Altos Hills, California. There, veterinary students are required to take a two-unit course in veterinary dentistry. We are fortunate to have the cooperation and use of the facilities of the Dental Hygiene department at the College to teach this course. The melding of accepted dental hygiene techniques with veterinary medicine advances the art of veterinary dentistry.

I would like to thank all the technicians with whom I have had the pleasure to work in my veterinary dental practice: Jan Yarslov, Gina Gros de Mange, Karen Thomson, David Kwoka, and Loretto Jaca. Thanks go to Karl Peter, DVM, Dipl ABVP, who is the director of the Veterinary Technology program at Foothill College and was helpful in the preliminary planning of this text. Credit should also go to the Foothill College Veterinary Technician students who helped with review: Pamela Hertz, Vicky Impett, Sacheen Koehn, Rebecca Lederer, Jo Lewis, Jennifer Lomb, Carol Oda, and Eliza Saclolo. Last, but not least, thanks to Carol Weldin, RDH, for her review of the periodontal sections of the text and her dedication to the advancement of veterinary dental education.

The contributors to this text, Laurie Holmstrom, Dr. Meghan Richey, Dr. Charles McGrath, and Dr. Robert Wiggs, contributed greatly to the successful completion of this text. Their efforts are sincerely appreciated.

Each chapter contains study questions in the form of work sheets. The answers to the work sheets are available on the Internet. Interested parties may E-mail Dr. Steven E. Holmstrom, Toothvet@aol.com. Comments and suggestions for future additions of this text should be addressed to the author at the above address.

STEVEN E. HOLMSTROM, DVM

Contents

VETERINARY DENTISTRY
for the Technician & Office Staff

1

Introduction

WHY VETERINARY DENTISTRY?

Just like humans need dental care, animals require veterinary dental care to maintain overall health. In addition to the discomfort caused by dental disease, the associated disease processes may cause systemic problems. The most common condition seen in general veterinary practice in dogs and cats over seven years of age is oral disease.

DENTAL ANATOMY AND DENTAL TERMINOLOGY

Communication in veterinary dentistry is as important as communication in veterinary medicine. Medical records and charts must be annotated. Dental terminology differs from that of veterinary medicine because the focus is on the teeth and their relationship to each other and the mouth.

GENERAL ANATOMY

To be able to recognize oral disease, technicians must first understand oral health. After establishing this baseline, technicians can recognize the changes that occur as oral disease progresses. Another reason that understanding normal anatomy is so important is that it helps veterinarians and technicians select the appropriate technique to use to prevent and treat disease. For example, without knowing the number of roots that tooth has, the practitioner could not extract a tooth.

Types of Heads

Three types of skulls are common: mesaticephalic, brachycephalic, and dolichocephalic. These words have a common root, *cephalic*, which means head.

Mesaticephalic

Mesatic means medium. Mesaticephalic is the most common head type. Poodles, corgis, German shepherds, Labrador retrievers, and domestic shorthair cats are typical examples (Fig. 1-1).

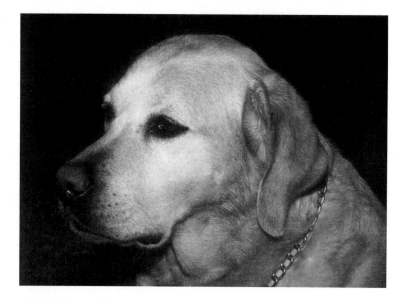

FIGURE 1-1 The Labrador retriever has a mesaticephalic head shape.

Brachycephalic

Brachy means short. Brachycephalic animals have short, wide heads. This character-
istic commonly results in crowded and rotated premolar teeth, a condition that may
lead to periodontal disease. Boxers, pugs, bulldogs, and Persian cats are common examples of the brachycephalic type (Fig. 1-2).

Dolichocephalic

Dolicho means long. Dolichocephalic animals have long, narrow heads. Collies,
greyhounds, borzois, and seal point Siamese cats are common examples of this
type (Fig. 1-3).

Maxilla

The upper jaw, called the *maxilla,* is made up of many bones (Fig. 1-4). The incisal
and maxillary bones hold the teeth. The roof of the mouth comprises the hard and
soft palates. The hard palate is the portion of the roof of the mouth that consists of
hard bone. The hard palate is covered with a mucous membrane that has irregular
ridges, called the *rugae palatinae.* The incisive papilla lies behind the central incisors.
The nasopalatine ducts exit on each side of the incisive papilla. The soft palate is the
posterior portion of the roof of the mouth, which does not have underlying bone.
This portion separates the oral cavity from the pharynx, which leads to the nasal
cavity. Close observation reveals that the teeth are surrounded by the gingiva. The
area where the two jaws join in the back of the oral cavity is known as the *fauca.*

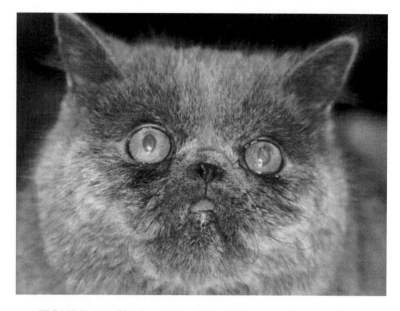

FIGURE 1-2 The Persian cat has a brachycephalic head shape.

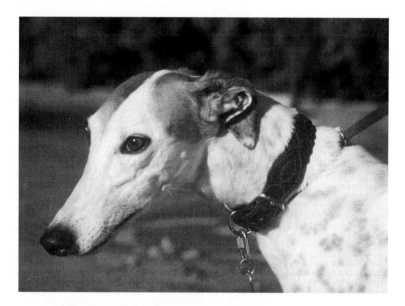

FIGURE 1-3 The greyhound has a dolichocephalic head shape.

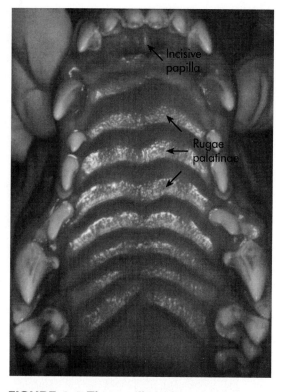

FIGURE 1-4 The maxilla is the upper jaw; note the incisive papilla and rugae, normal features in the maxilla.

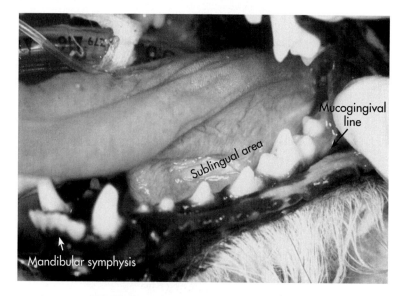

FIGURE 1-5 The mandible is the lower jaw.

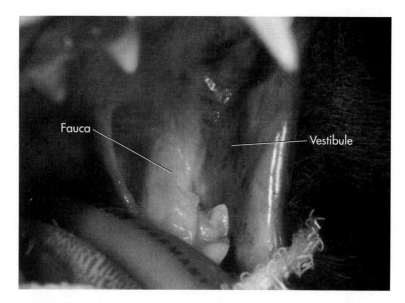

Fauca

Vestibule

FIGURE 1-6 The vestibule is the area between the cheeks and teeth.

Mandible

The lower jaw is known as the *mandible* (Fig. 1-5). It is connected to the maxilla by a hinge joint called the *temporomandibular joint,* or *TMJ.* The two mandibles are fused together at the mandibular symphysis. The tongue lies between the two mandibles, and the structures and surfaces beneath the tongue are referred to as *sublingual.* The mandible is covered ventrally by muscle and skin. The oral cavity is covered with a mucous membrane, which becomes the gingiva at the mucogingival line.

Cheeks and Lips

The mucous membrane, or oral mucosa, is the tissue that forms the lining of most of the oral cavity outside the mucogingival line. The oral mucosa ends at the lips. The vestibule of the oral cavity is the part between the cheeks or lips and the alveolar ridge (Fig. 1-6).

TOOTH ANATOMY

The puppy has 28 teeth, whereas the adult dog has 42 teeth. The kitten has 26 teeth, whereas the adult cat has 30 teeth.

External Tooth

The tooth may be divided into the crown, neck, and root (Fig. 1-7). The tip of the crown is known as the *cusp.* The crown is covered with enamel, the hardest substance in the body. It will survive normal use and even some abuse without problems. How-

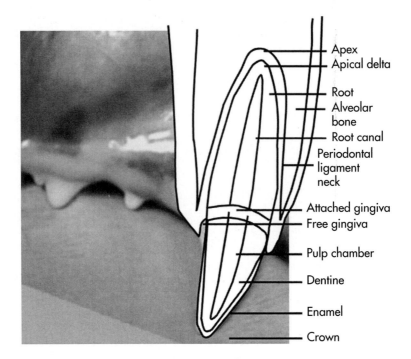

FIGURE 1-7 Dental anatomy.

ever, it may fracture in patients who chew bones and other hard substances. Normally, enamel is present only above the gumline. Enamel is produced by cells called *ameloblasts* as the tooth is developing. Where the enamel thins close to the gumline, many teeth have a slight indentation. This indentation is known as the *neck*. Underneath the gumline is the root. The deepest part of the root is known as the *apex*. [*Apex. The terminal portion of the root.*] At the apex, blood vessels and nerves enter the tooth through a series of small channels known as the *apical delta* or through larger canals known as the *apical foramen*. [*Apical delta. The diverging branches of the root canal at the apical end of the tooth root.*] [*Apical foramen. The opening(s) in the apex of the root through which nerves and vessels pass into the root canal.*] The cusp is the tip or pointed prominence on the occlusal surface of the crown.

Internal Tooth

The bulk of the tooth consists of dentine, or dentin. Both spellings are correct and synonymous. Dentine is produced by odontoblasts, which are cells that line the pulp chamber. Throughout the life of the tooth the odontoblast continues to produce dentine. The innermost portion of the tooth is the pulp chamber. As previously mentioned, the pulp chamber is lined by odontoblasts. The remainder of the pulp chamber consists of nerves, blood vessels, and a variety of different types of cells and fibrous tissue. The root canal is the portion of the pulp chamber below the gumline. The apex of the tooth is the portion deepest in the socket (or alveolus). The apex contains small channels through which blood vessels and nerves enter and exit.

Gingiva

Attached gingiva is made up of epithelial tissue that is harder and more tightly attached to supportive structures than other tissue in the oral cavity. Gingiva is therefore able to withstand the forces of chewing. This hardening is known as *keratinization*. Free gingiva is the portion of the gingiva that is not directly attached to the tooth or supporting structure. A slight groove exists between the free and attached gingiva, which is known as the *free gingival groove*. The area between the free gingiva and the tooth is known as the *sulcus* when healthy and without a space. A space between the gingiva and tooth is called a *pocket*. Pockets are considered diseased tissue when periodontal disease is present.

Alveolar Mucosa

The alveolar mucosa is the less densely keratinized gingival tissue covering the bone. Its decreased keratinization increases the susceptibility of the tissue to trauma caused by chewing.

Attachment Apparatus

The attachment apparatus comprises the structures that support the tooth. The tooth is held in place in the alveolus, or socket, by the periodontal ligament. *[Alveolus. The cavity or socket in either jawbone that surrounds and supports the root of the tooth.]* Cementum, a material that can repair itself if damaged, attaches the periodontal ligament to the tooth. The periodontal ligament is a fibrous structure attached to the tooth/cementum and bone by Sharpey's fibers. These fibers are interlaced in cementum and bone. The alveolar bone is the bone of the upper jaw (maxilla) or lower jaw (mandible) in which the tooth rests. *[Alveolar bone. Cancellous bone directly surrounding the tooth roots.] [Cementum. A specialized calcified connective tissue covering the root surface and serving as attachment for the periodontal ligament from the bone to the tooth.]*

DENTAL FORMULA FOR THE PUPPY

The puppy is born without teeth. Primary ("baby," or deciduous) canine dentition consists of 28 teeth. The primary incisors normally erupt at approximately 3 to 4 weeks of age, the canines at 3 weeks, and the primary premolars from 4 to 12 weeks of age. The age at which the teeth erupt varies among breed lines. On each side, upper and lower, the adult dog has three incisors, one canine, and three premolars. Puppies do not have primary molars. The dental formula for the puppy is listed as follows:

$$2 \times (3/3\,i,\, 1/1\,c,\, 3/3\,p) = 28.$$

Generally, primary teeth fall out (exfoliate) 1 to 2 weeks before the eruption of adult teeth. What triggers a tooth to exfoliate is not fully understood. One theory is that as the adult tooth develops, it puts pressure on the primary tooth, stimulating a resorptive process. Once the tooth root is resorbed, the crown loosens from the gingival attachment and falls off.

DENTAL FORMULA FOR THE ADULT DOG

The secondary (adult) canine dental formula on each side of the mouth, upper and lower, consists of three incisors, one canine, and four premolars. On each side, the upper jaw has two molars and the lower jaw has three molars. The incisors are used for gnawing and grooming. The canine teeth are used for holding and tearing. The arrangement of the premolars, which are used for cutting and breaking up food, resembles pinking shears. The molars are used for grinding. The adult incisor teeth erupt at 3 to 5 months of age, the canine and premolar teeth at 4 to 6 months, and the molars at 5 to 7 months. The dental formula for the adult dog is as follows:

$$2 \times (3/3\text{I}, 1/1\text{C}, 4/4\text{P}, 2/3\text{M}) = 42$$

DENTAL FORMULA FOR THE KITTEN

The kitten's dentition is similar to that of the puppy except that two, rather than three, primary premolars are present in the lower jaw. The kitten's primary teeth erupt earlier than those of the puppy. The incisors erupt at 2 to 3 weeks of age. The canines erupt at 3 to 4 weeks of age, and the premolars at 3 to 6 weeks of age. The dental formula for a kitten is listed as follows:

$$2 \times (3/3 \text{ i}, 1/1 \text{ c}, 3/2\text{p}) = 26$$

DENTAL FORMULA FOR THE ADULT CAT

On each side of the mouth, upper and lower, the adult cat has three incisors, one canine, and one molar. On each side the cat has three premolars on the upper jaw and two premolars on the lower jaw. The adult incisors erupt at 3 to 4 months of age, the canines at 4 to 5 months of age, premolars at 4 to 6 months of age, and molars at 4 to 5 months of age. The dental formula for the adult cat is as follows:

$$2 \times (3/3 \text{ I}, 1/1 \text{ C}, 3/2\text{P}, 1/1\text{M}) = 30$$

ROOT STRUCTURE OF THE ADULT DOG

An understanding of root structure is important. When extracting teeth (with a few exceptions discussed later), all roots should be removed to prevent further complications. To remove all the roots, the technician must know the number of roots and understand the anatomy. In the dog the incisors, canines, first premolar, and mandibular third molar have one root each. The maxillary second and third premolars; the mandibular second, third, and fourth premolars; and the mandibular first and second molars have two roots. The maxillary fourth premolar, first molar, and second molar have three roots each. One key to remembering the number of roots is to recall that the mandible does not have any three-rooted teeth (Figs. 1-8 and 1-9).

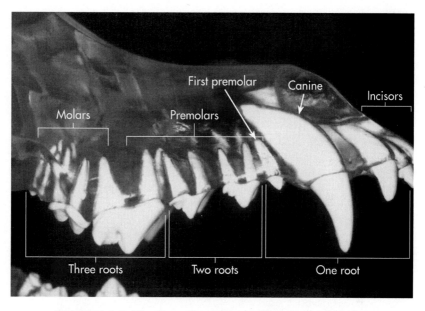

FIGURE 1-8 Numbers of roots in maxillary teeth of the dog.

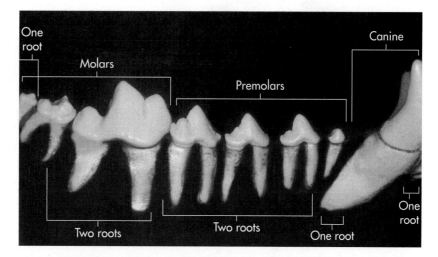

FIGURE 1-9 Numbers of roots in mandibular teeth of the dog.

ROOT STRUCTURE OF THE ADULT CAT

In the cat the incisors, canines, and maxillary second premolar have one root each. The maxillary third premolars, mandibular third and fourth premolars, and mandibular first molar have two roots. The maxillary fourth premolar has three roots. The number of roots in the maxillary first molar varies from one to three roots, which are usually fused together (Figs. 1-10 and 1-11).

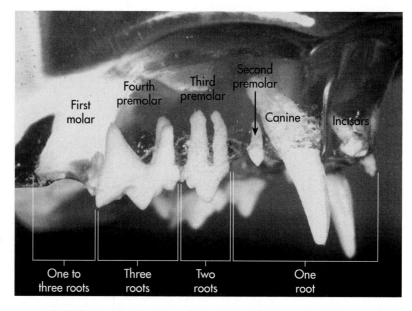

FIGURE 1-10 Numbers of roots in maxillary teeth of the cat.

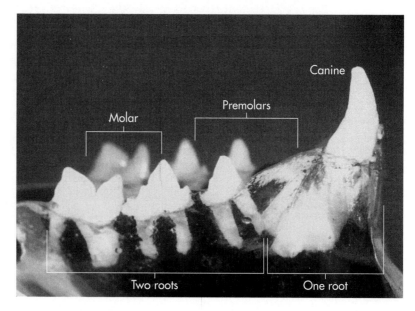

FIGURE 1-11 Numbers of roots in mandibular teeth of the cat.

FURCATION

The furcation is the area where the roots join the crown. In two rooted teeth, it is known as a *bifurcation;* in three rooted teeth, a *trifurcation.*

NOMENCLATURE

The term *nomenclature* is derived from the words "name" and "to call."

POSITIONAL TERMINOLOGY

The reference point for anatomic terms in the mouth is the teeth. The term *labial* indicates the direction toward the outside of the teeth, usually toward the lips. Similarly, *buccal* indicates the direction toward the outside of the teeth, usually toward the cheeks. *Palatal* and *lingual* refer to the direction toward the inside of the tooth—palatal for the maxillary and lingual for the mandibular. Although these terms are often used interchangeably, they are properly used specifically for upper and lower dentition, respectively. If a line is drawn along the dental arch and a mark is placed representing the center of the line between the first incisors, mesial is the side of the tooth closest to the center of the line and distal is the portion farthest from the center of the line (Fig. 1-12).

Line Angles

Line angles represent the "corners" of the tooth. The mesial buccal line angle is the area where the mesial and buccal surfaces join. Likewise, the buccal distal line angle joins the distal and buccal walls. The distal lingual and lingual mesial serve as similar reference points. Line angles and walls are important in describing fractures and tooth defects.

Coronal-Apical Directions

Coronal refers to the direction toward the crown, and *apical* means toward the apex of the tooth. For example, a fracture at the tip of the crown could also be described as a fracture in the coronal third of the tooth.

Between Teeth

The area in between the teeth is known as the *interproximal area.*

OCCLUSION

Occlusion refers to the way the teeth fit together. Humans have true occlusal surfaces, in which the premolars and molars directly oppose each other. Chewing takes place

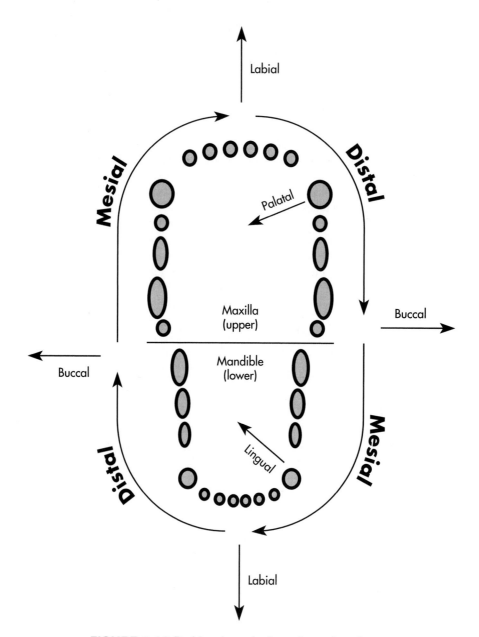

FIGURE 1-12 Positional terminology: the oral road map.

on a flat surface. Dogs and cats have sectorial occlusion, whereby chewing occurs on the sides of the teeth.

ANATOMIC AND TRIADAN NUMBERING SYSTEMS

In human dentistry the universal nomenclature system is standard. In this system the numbering starts with the upper right third molar (#1) and proceeds around the arch to #16. The lower left third molar is #17, and counting proceeds around the arch to the lower right third molar, #32. *[Arch, dental. The dentition and alveolar ridge of either the maxilla or the mandible; sometimes called either the upper or lower arch.]*

Because the veterinary profession treats a variety of species with different numbers of teeth, use of the universal system is impractical; it would result in the same tooth being identified by a different number depending on the animal. For that reason the veterinary profession has adopted the anatomic and triadan numbering systems. By using the anatomic or triadan system, veterinary staff members can easily annotate medical records. Currently, both the anatomic and triadan systems are acceptable. Each system has advantages and disadvantages.

Anatomic System

The first thing to know with the anatomic system is tooth type. The beginning of this chapter contained a review of the types and functions of teeth. The first letter of the tooth is used to identify the tooth type.

Incisors = I
The incisors are identified by the capital letter *I*. When writing the tooth type on ruled paper, the veterinary staff member should generally write the letter on the line. A lowercase letter *i* should be used in reference to a primary tooth. The incisor located closest to the center of the mouth is incisor #1, incisor #2 is the intermediate incisor, and incisor #3 is the lateral incisor. The central right maxillary incisor is I^1. The central left mandibular incisor is $_1I$.

Canines = C
The adult canine teeth are identified by the capital letter *C*. The primary canine tooth is indicated by the lowercase letter *c*. A quadrant is one quarter, and the mouth has four quadrants: upper right, upper left, lower left, and lower right. Because only one canine tooth is present in each quadrant, only the number *1* is used. The left mandibular canine is known as $_1C$. The right maxillary canine tooth is known as C^1.

Premolars = P
The premolars are represented by the capital letter *P*. Primary premolar teeth are represented by a lowercase *p*. In the dog the premolars are numbered sequentially beginning with *1* and moving back in the mouth. Because the cat does not have a first premolar in the maxilla (upper jaw) or a first or second premolar in the mandible (lower jaw), premolar numbering starts with *2* in the maxilla and *3* in the

mandible. The left maxillary fourth premolar is called ^{4}P, and the right mandibular fourth premolar is called P_4. The cat does not have ^{1}P, P^1, $_1$P, $_2$P, P$_1$, and P$_2$.

Molars = M

The molars are indicated by the letter *M*. Remember that no primary molars exist. The first molar is indicated by *1,* and successive molars by *2* and *3* if present. The right maxillary first molar is M^1. The left mandibular first molar is $_1$M.

To indicate the side of the mouth where the tooth is, a number representing the tooth is written on the left side of the letter for the left side of the patient's mouth or on the right side of the letter for the right side of the patient's mouth. A helpful way to remember this convention is as follows: left side of patient, left side of letter; right side of patient, right side of letter.

The maxillary (upper) teeth are indicated as a superscript number. The mandibular teeth are indicated as a subscript number.

Primary (deciduous) teeth

The primary teeth are indicated by lowercase letters. A lowercase *i* indicates a primary incisor, a lowercase *c* a canine, and *p* a premolar.

Shortcut

A shortcut in the notation of multiple teeth is to indicate the tooth numbers as a chain. For example, ^{321}I^{123} indicates all the maxillary incisors.

Modification for alphanumeric computers

The use of computers in veterinary medicine is increasing. For the purposes of estimating and invoicing, codes can be created to indicate various types of treatment of individual teeth. The letter *U* is used for upper teeth, and *L* is used for lower teeth. For example, one code might be RCULC (**R**oot **C**anal **U**pper **L**eft **C**anine) to indicate a root canal performed on the upper left canine tooth. Similarly, DXLP4 (**De**ntal e**X**traction **L**ower **P**remolar) might indicate an extraction of the lower right fourth premolar.

Advantages

The primary advantage of the anatomic system is that it is easy to remember because it uses anatomic terms that most people already know. Also, by using the previously described shortcut, veterinary staff members can refer to many teeth at once.

Disadvantages

One disadvantage of this system is that it is more time-consuming than the triadan system, which will be discussed next. Although shorter than "left maxillary canine," the words "one superscript C" still take more time to say than the numbers of the triadan system. Moreover, not all computers are alphanumeric. Some computer systems accept only numbers. Because the creation of codes would be difficult with this type of computer, the triadan system is particularly useful.

Triadan System

The many numbers in the triadan system make it seem confusing at first (Table 1-1). Despite its appearance, the triadan system is quite simple once the code is memorized. The triadan system uses three numbers. The first number identifies the quadrant (remember that there are four) of the mouth. The second and third numbers identify the tooth, which is always represented by two numbers.

Quadrant

The quadrants are identified as *1* for right maxillary, *2* for left maxillary, *3* for left mandibular, and *4* for right mandibular. The quadrant is indicated by the first of three numbers (Fig. 1-13).

TABLE 1-1
Anatomic vs. Triadan

	Anatomic	Triadan
Computers	Will not work with nonalphanumeric types	Works with both types
Shortcut	Can identify many teeth of the same type	Identifies each tooth separately
Ease of use	Familiar terms, easy to remember	Not intuitive, must be memorized

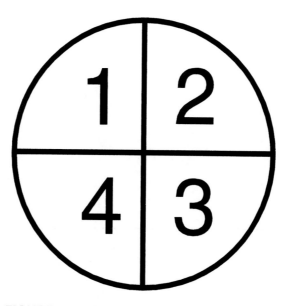

FIGURE 1-13 Quadrants used in the triadan system.

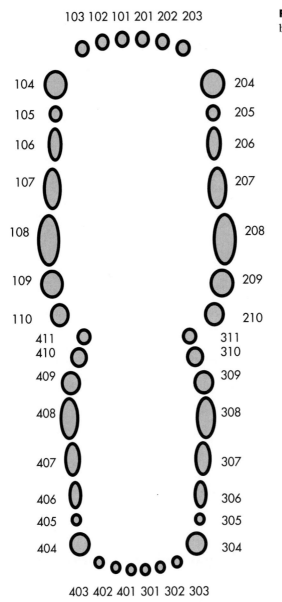

103 102 101 201 202 203

FIGURE 1-14 Triadan dental numbering system in the dog.

403 402 401 301 302 303

Tooth

The numbering of the teeth begins in the front of the mouth. The central incisor is identified as *tooth 01*, the intermediate incisor as *02*, the lateral (or corner) incisor as *03*, the canine as *04*, the first premolar as *05*, and the first molar as *09*. Remember, in the triadan system the type of tooth is *always* identified by two numbers. Combined with the quadrant, there are three numbers. For example, the left maxillary canine tooth is identified as *204*. The right maxillary fourth premolar is identified as *108*, the left mandibular first molar as *309*, and the right mandibular central incisor as *401* (Figs. 1-14 and 1-15).

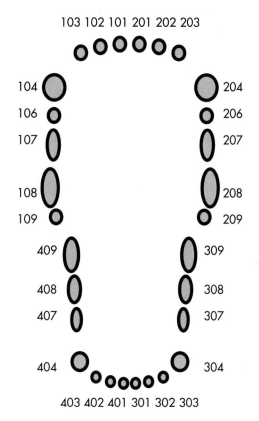

103 102 101 201 202 203

104
106
107
108
109

204
206
207
208
209

409
408
407

309
308
307

404
403 402 401 301 302 303
304

FIGURE 1-15 Triadan dental numbering system in the cat.

Rule of 4 and 9

For species that have fewer teeth, the rule of 4 and 9 has been developed. This rule states that the canine tooth is always designated by *04* and the first molar by *09*. Teeth are counted from 01 to 05. The first molar is counted as 09, and then the count goes backward, with the fourth premolar being 08 and the third premolar being 07, just as it is in the dog. This convention allows identical teeth to have identical numbers in different species and decreases confusion.

Primary (deciduous) teeth

In the young patient, primary teeth are identified as being in quadrants 5 for the right maxillary (upper), 6 for the left maxillary (upper), 7 for the left mandibular (lower), and 8 for the right mandibular (lower).

Advantages

The primary advantage of the triadan system is that it can be used with nonalphanumeric computers. Secondly, referring to the tooth type as "one-o-one" for the right maxillary first incisor or "three eleven" for the left mandibular third molar is convenient.

Disadvantage

The disadvantage of the triadan system is that it is not intuitive. The technician must know the code to understand which tooth is being identified. Although its popularity has increased in recent years, the triadan system is not as universal or easy to learn as the anatomic system.

DENTAL CHART FOR THE DOG

A dental chart may be used to keep a visual record of the patient's oral health status (Fig. 1-16). The teeth are oriented to the viewer, who is facing the patient. The patient's right side is indicated on the left side of the chart, and the patient's left side is on the right side of the chart. The first row of teeth represents the labial/buccal

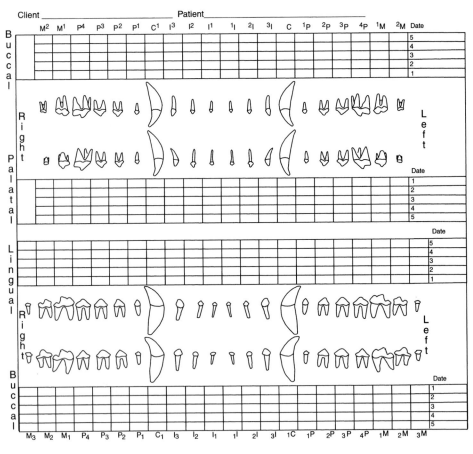

FIGURE 1-16 Canine dental chart.

(outside) of the maxillary (upper) teeth. The second row of teeth represents the palatal (inside) of the maxillary teeth. The third row of teeth represents the lingual (inside) of the mandibular (lower) teeth. The lowest row of teeth represents the labial/buccal (outside) of the mandibular (lower) teeth. The boxes indicate the depth of the sulcus, or pocket, at the time of successive dental procedures. The first charted depth is indicated in the row closest to the tooth (date #1). Successive procedures are noted in the next rows.

DENTAL CHART FOR THE CAT

Except for the number of teeth, the dental chart for the cat is identical to that of the dog (Fig. 1-17).

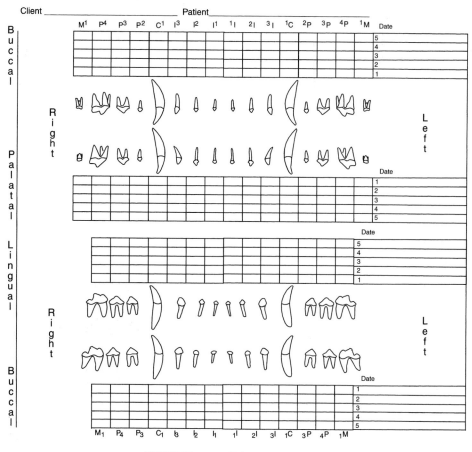

FIGURE 1-17 Feline dental chart.

Worksheet

STUDENT NAME:_____

1. The most common condition in cats over 7 years of age is

   _____.

2. Dental terminology is different from veterinary medical terminology in that the focus is on the teeth themselves and the relationship of the _____ to other teeth.

3. For example, practitioners could not extract a tooth without knowing the number of _____ that the tooth has.

4. The area where the two jaws join in the oral cavity is known as the _____.

5. The puppy has _____ teeth, whereas the adult dog has _____ teeth.

6. _____ is the hardest substance in the body and is fairly resistant to stains.

7. Dentine is produced by _____, which are cells that line the pulp chamber.

8. The area between the free gingiva and the tooth is known as the _____ in healthy animals when there is no space between the gingiva and tooth and a _____ when there is space.

9. The tooth is held in place in the alveolus or socket by the

   _____ _____.

10. The dental formula for the adult dog is: _____.

11. The dental formula for the adult cat is: _____.

12. The following maxillary teeth have one root in the dog (use triadan or anatomic system): _____.

13. The following mandibular teeth have two roots in the dog (use triadan or anatomic system): _____.

14. The following maxillary teeth have three roots in the dog (use triadan or anatomic system): _____.

15. The following maxillary teeth have three roots in the cat (use triadan or anatomic system): _____.

16. The primary teeth are indicated by _____ _____ letters.

17. In the triadan system, adult quadrants are identified as _____ for right maxillary, _____ for left maxillary, _____ for left mandibular, and _____ for right mandibular. The quadrant is indicated as the first of three numbers.

18. The central incisor is identified as tooth _____, the intermediate incisor is identified as tooth _____, the lateral (or corner) incisor is identified as tooth _____, the canine as _____, and first premolar as _____.

19. The rule of 4 and 9 states that 04 is always the _____ tooth and the _____ _____ is always tooth 09.

20. The left maxillary first premolar in the dog would be listed as tooth # _____, whereas the right mandibular third premolar in the cat would be listed as tooth # _____.

2

The Oral Examination and Disease Recognition

This chapter is devoted to an overview of the oral examination and the recognition of veterinary dental disease. Because it is an overview, it does not provide in-depth coverage of specific aspects of treatment. The treatment of veterinary dental conditions will be covered in subsequent chapters.

All the members of the veterinary office staff play important parts in health care. Although the diagnosis of disease should be left to the veterinarian, the technician and other staff members can assist the veterinarian by recognizing conditions that appear abnormal and alerting the veterinarian to them. This chapter discusses various disease conditions that staff members may observe.

ORAL EXAMINATION

The duties of veterinarians and their staff are described in the practice acts of each state. Because state law varies, veterinary staff members should refer to the specific practice acts of the state in which they are employed. However, some generalities apply. The oral examination should always be conducted in a systematic manner. In many states, it is legal for the registered veterinary technician to induce anesthesia under orders of a licensed veterinarian. The placement of the endotracheal tube is a good opportunity for visualization of the pharynx, tonsils, and tongue (Fig. 2-1). While scaling and polishing the teeth, the technician can closely observe the tooth surface and gingiva. The technician should always note any abnormalities and report them to the doctor.

NORMAL OCCLUSION

Normal occlusion in dogs and cats is a scissors bite, in which the mandibular (lower) teeth come into contact with the palatal side (inside) of the maxillary (upper) teeth (Figs. 2-2 and 2-3). Normally the cusp of the mandibular incisors rests on a ledge on the palatal side of the maxillary incisors known as the *cingulum*. The mandibular

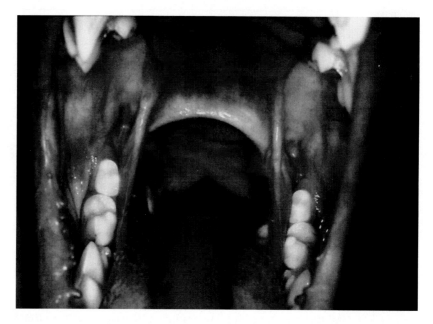

FIGURE 2-1 The process of intubation provides a good opportunity for examination deep in the oral cavity.

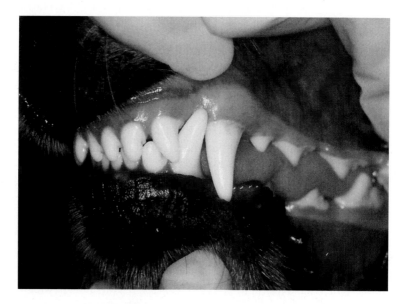

FIGURE 2-2 Normal canine occlusion.

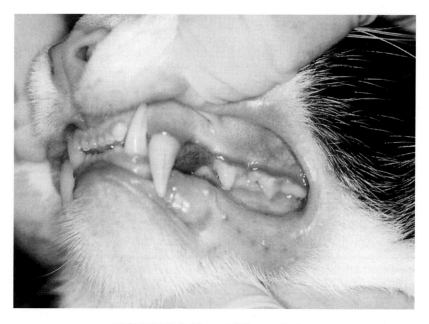

FIGURE 2-3 Normal feline occlusion.

canines fit in the diastema (space) between the lateral incisor and maxillary canines. *[Diastema. The space between two adjacent teeth that are not in contact with each other in an arch.]* The cusp of the mandibular first premolar fits midway between the maxillary canine and first premolar. The remainder of the premolars are intermeshed in a similar fashion, the lower teeth approximately one-half a tooth in front of their maxillary counterparts.

SPECIALTIES OF DENTISTRY

In the past, veterinarians were expected to treat all animals for any conditions they might have. Veterinary medicine has since become more sophisticated; with the advancement of knowledge, no veterinarian can perform all facets of veterinary medicine. Consequently, the field is now increasingly specialized. In fact, human dentistry is subdivided into specialties (Table 2-1), a phenomenon that is becoming increasingly common in veterinary dentistry as well. The more a practitioner performs a particular skill, the better the practitioner becomes. Therefore treatment of advanced periodontal disease, fractured teeth, and orthodontic conditions may not be in the patient's best interest when the practitioner performs these procedures only occasionally. Furthermore, preparing the practice for the occasional specialized procedure requires considerable expense, training, and time. In this case, the "win-win" solution is referral.

TABLE 2-1 Dental Disciplines

Branch of dentistry	Area of specialization
Endodontics	Treatment of diseases that affect the tooth pulp and apical periodontal tissues
Exodontics	Extraction of teeth and related procedures
Oral surgery	Surgery of the oral cavity
Orthodontics	Guidance and correction of malocclusion of the juvenile teeth and adult tooth positioning
Periodontics	Study and treatment of diseases of the tooth-supporting tissues
Prosthodontics	Construction of appliances designed to replace missing teeth and/or other adjacent structures
Restorative/operative dentistry	Restoration of form and function of teeth

ORAL DISEASES AND DENTAL SPECIALTIES

Because of the variety of disease conditions, a variety of dental specialties exists. Pedodontics is the treatment of dental disease in the puppy and kitten. Orthodontics is the treatment of disease related to the way the teeth fit together. Periodontics is the treatment of conditions in the surrounding tooth structure (*perio* means around, and *dontics* means tooth). Prosthodontics involves the process of restoring the tooth to normal health. *Endodontics* means "inside the tooth." Oral medicine deals with the effects of cancer and other medical conditions on the mouth.

Pedodontics

Puppies and kittens exhibit a variety of dental conditions, both genetic (inherited) and acquired.

Missing teeth

Anodontia refers to the absence of teeth. Teeth may be missing because they never developed in the first place, are slow to erupt, or were present and fell out. Dental radiographs must be taken to evaluate the area of the missing tooth. In dental charts a circle around the tooth indicates that it is missing. The patient in Fig. 2-4 is a 6-month-old Lhasa apso; neither the primary nor the adult teeth have erupted. Protrusions in the mucous membrane indicate the presence of teeth, possibly the maxillary lateral primary incisors ($^3i^3$, 503, 603), that may be close to erupting.

A radiograph should be taken to evaluate the oral structure for missing teeth (see Chapter 11 for technique). The radiograph indicates whether the root is miss-

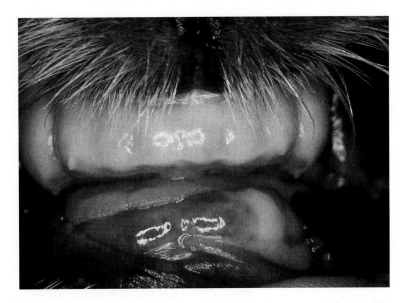

FIGURE 2-4 A 6-month-old Lhasa apso showing a lack of primary or adult teeth. The primary lateral incisors may be starting to erupt.

ing or retained. The absence of the root may be inherited or the result of trauma. In the patient shown in Fig. 2-4, a Lhasa apso, most of the primary incisors are missing.

Persistent primary teeth

Persistent primary (also called *retained, deciduous,* or *baby*) teeth may cause orthodontic and periodontic abnormalities. Extraction of these teeth may help prevent such complications. In the patient shown in Fig. 2-5 the primary tooth is displacing the maxillary canine. In addition to causing the possible displacement of the adult canine, the abnormal periodontal border may cause periodontal disease resulting from plaque being trapped between the primary and adult teeth. The general rule applies: There is no room for two teeth of the same type in the same mouth at the same time. Unless they are extremely loose, retained primary teeth should be extracted as soon as possible after the adult tooth starts to erupt. The dental chart symbol is "RD." The patient in Fig. 2-5 has a persistent left maxillary canine (^{1}c, 604), which should be extracted.

The term *interceptive orthodontics* describes the process of extracting primary teeth to prevent orthodontic malocclusions. Extraction of these teeth does not cause the jaw to grow correctly or longer. Rather, it removes any possible obstruction to the full development of the jaw. Normally the primary mandibular (lower) canine occludes mesial to the primary maxillary (upper) canine. In this case the mandibular primary canine is "trapped" by the maxillary primary canine. Further forward growth of the

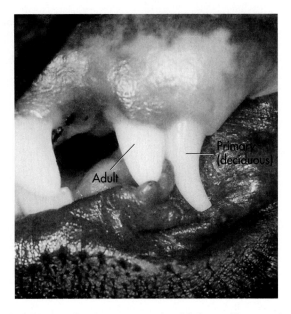

FIGURE 2-5 Persistent or retained left maxillary canine.

mandible cannot occur. To be effective, this type of interceptive orthodontic treatment should be performed before the patient reaches 12 weeks of age, preferably much earlier. The dental chart symbol is "IOD" for deciduous (primary) teeth or "IOP" for permanent (adult) teeth. A list of treatment codes can be found at the end of the chapter.

Cranial mandibular osteodystrophy

Cranial mandibular osteodystrophy is an inherited condition that occurs primarily in West Highland white terriers and occasionally in other breeds. Nonneoplastic bone forms in the region of the temporomandibular joint and occasionally extends into the mandible. Patients with cranial mandibular osteodystrophy are treated symptomatically for pain, which usually lessens as the patient gets older. The medical record abbreviation for this condition is "CMO." Fig. 2-6 shows increased density in the lower right portion of the photograph, which represents nonneoplastic bone production in the region of the temporomandibular joint.

Fractured primary teeth

Fractured primary teeth occur fairly frequently. They may be caused by running into objects, catching rocks or other hard substances, or overzealous playing of games such as tug-of-war. If left untreated, fractured primary teeth may result in abscessation and formation of stoma (fistula), which can in turn cause a defect in enamel production known as *enamel hypoplasia*. The symbol for a fractured tooth is "FX." Fig. 2-7 shows a fractured left maxillary canine ([1]c, 604). Note the fistula formation

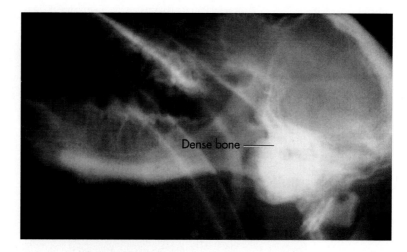

FIGURE 2-6 Cranial mandibular osteodystrophy.

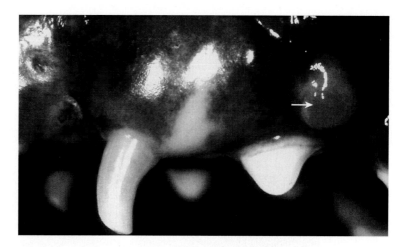

FIGURE 2-7 Fractured primary teeth.

(arrow) above the premolar as an extension of the fracture and subsequent abscess. This tooth should be extracted.

Supernumerary teeth

Supernumerary teeth are primarily incisors, although all types of teeth may be supernumerary. One problem that supernumerary teeth may cause is crowding. The chart symbol for supernumerary tooth is "SN," with the additional tooth drawn where it appears. The patient in Fig. 2-8 has a supernumerary left mandibular fourth premolar ($_4$P, 308).

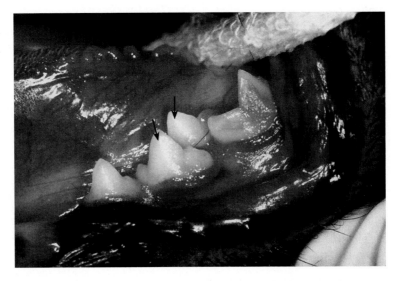

FIGURE 2-8 Supernumerary mandibular fourth premolars in a cat.

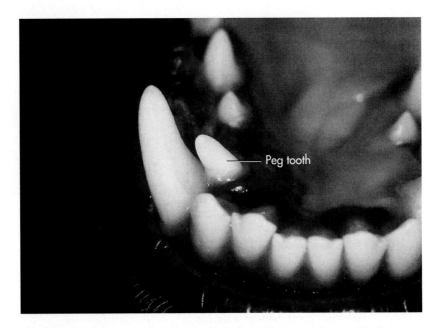

FIGURE 2-9 Mandibular peg tooth located lingual to the right mandibular canine.

Peg teeth

Peg teeth are abnormally formed supernumerary teeth. They generally occur in the canine and incisor regions. The treatment is extraction. The patient in Fig. 2-9 has a peg tooth located lingual to the right mandibular canine (C_1, 404).

Third set of teeth

Supernumerary teeth may also result from the formation of a third set of teeth. The primary teeth of the patient in Fig. 2-10 fell out at the normal time. The outermost row of teeth are adult teeth. A supernumerary third row of teeth is present in this patient. The innermost row of teeth was extracted.

Fused and gemini teeth

Fusion is the joining of two developing teeth that have different tooth buds. A gemini tooth is one in which a tooth bud has partially divided in the attempt to form two teeth. The left central incisor (^{1}I, 201) in Fig. 2-11 is a gemini tooth.

Orthodontic Disease

Orthodontic disease is oral disease caused by the malalignment of teeth.

Class I malocclusion

Patients with Class I malocclusion have overall normal occlusions except that one or more teeth are out of alignment. Class I malocclusion occurs in several disease conditions. The abbreviation for a Class I malocclusion is "CI0."

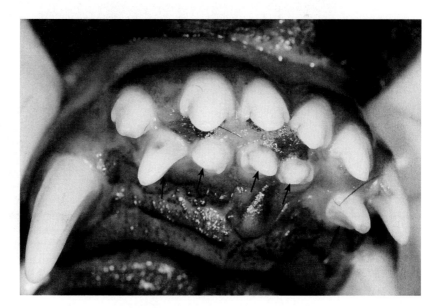

FIGURE 2-10 Third set of teeth in a dog.

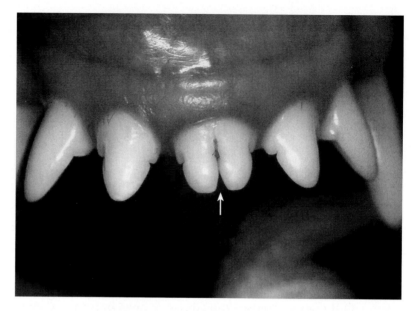

FIGURE 2-11 Gemini left central incisor.

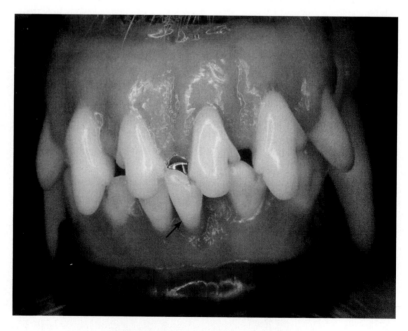

FIGURE 2-12 Anterior cross-bite.

Anterior cross-bite

An anterior cross-bite is a normal occlusion except that one or more of the incisors are malaligned. In the patient in Fig. 2-12 the maxillary central and intermediate incisors are displaced palatally and the mandibular central, intermediate, and lateral incisors are displaced labially. Untreated, these teeth (usually the mandibular incisors) may fall out because of chronic trauma. Several treatment options exist, including extraction of the malaligned teeth and placement of an orthodontic appliance to move the maxillary teeth labially and the mandibular teeth lingually. The left maxillary central incisor (^{1}I, 201) in Fig. 2-12 is occluding buccal to the corresponding maxillary incisors.

Posterior cross-bite

In posterior cross-bite, the maxillary premolars are lingual to the mandibular premolars or molars. The symbol is "PXB." The left mandibular first molar ($_1$M, 309) is occluding buccal to the left maxillary fourth premolar (^{4}P, 208) in Fig. 2-13.

Base-narrowed canines

Base-narrowed canines may be caused by a structural narrowing of the mandible or by the eruption of the canines in an overly upright position. The mandibular canines normally diverge from each other. Base-narrowed canines may cause in-

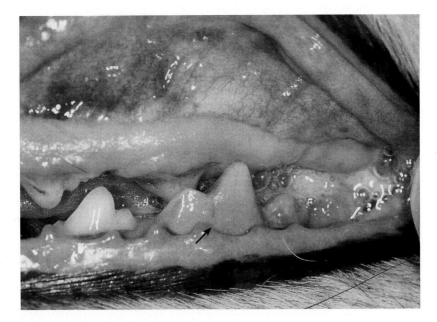

FIGURE 2-13 Posterior cross-bite causing left mandibular first molar *(arrow)* to occlude buccal to the maxillary fourth premolar.

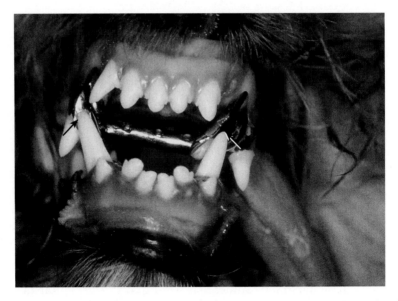

FIGURE 2-14 Base-narrowed canines *(arrows)* being treated with a telescoping incline plane.

dentation into and ulceration of the hard palate. The patient in Fig. 2-14 is being treated with a metal telescoping incline plane. As the mandibular canines ($_1C_1$, 304, 404) hit the plane, they are deflected buccally.

Spearing (lancing) canines
When the maxillary canines are tipped in a rostral position, they are trapped by the mandibular canines. This Class I orthodontic condition is known as *spearing canines.* Other terms that are sometimes used are *lancing* and *tusk teeth.* The condition appears to be genetic and is most prevalent in shelties and Persian cats. Treatment includes orthodontic correction and extraction. The cat in Fig. 2-15 has a spearing left maxillary canine (^1C, 204).

Spearing (lancing) lateral incisors
Spearing, or lancing, may also occur with the lateral incisors. Occasionally, this condition corrects itself. In Fig. 2-16 the left maxillary lateral incisor (^3I, 203) is spearing and rotated; the left maxillary central incisor (^1I, 201) is also displaced.

Class II Malocclusion
A Class II malocclusion occurs when the mandible is shorter than normal. This may cause the adult canines and incisors to penetrate the hard palate, and irritation and ulceration of the hard palate may result. The symbol for a Class II malocclusion is "C2O." The mandibular incisors ($_{321}I_{123}$, 301, 302, 303, 401, 402, 403) and canines ($_1C_1$, 304, 404) have indented the hard palate of the patient in Fig. 2-17.

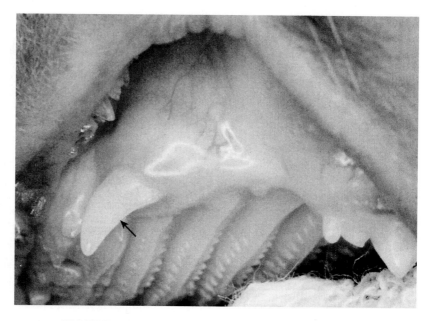

FIGURE 2-15 Spearing, or tusk, maxillary canine *(arrow)*.

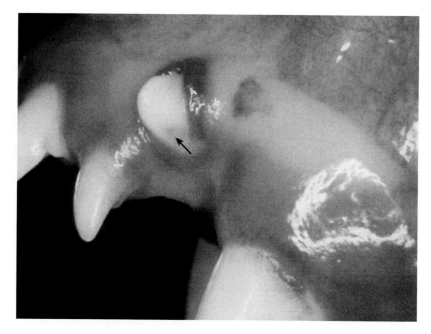

FIGURE 2-16 Spearing lateral maxillary incisor *(arrow)*.

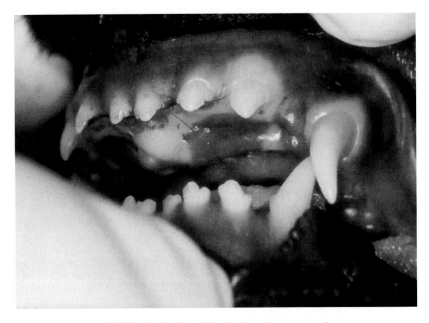

FIGURE 2-17 Class II occlusion in a young dog.

Class III Malocclusion
Mandibular prognathism

Class III malocclusion has several forms. It may be caused by the mandible being too long (mandibular prognathism). [Pro *means long*, gnath *means jaw*]. As a result, the mandibular incisors occlude labial to the maxillary incisors. With time this may cause excessive wear and injury to both teeth. The mandible may be "bowed," causing excess space between the premolars, known as excess *freeway space*. The longer mandible may cause severe wear as shown in Fig. 2-26. Another form of Class III malocclusion may be caused by the maxilla being too short. In this case, there may be associated crowding of the maxillary teeth. In Fig. 2-18 the left mandibular canine ($_1$C, 304) is occluding against the maxillary lateral incisor (^{3}I, 203).

Maxillary brachygnathism

The condition known as maxillary brachygnathism [brachy *means short*, gnath *means jaw*] is caused by a shortened maxilla. Typically, the maxillary teeth are rotated as a result of crowding. The lower jaw is normal length, as evidenced by the lack of tooth crowding. The mandible may be bowed, causing excess space between the upper and lower premolars. When charting, the veterinary technician should redraw the rotated tooth over the normal tooth position. The right mandibular canine is occluding labial to the maxillary lateral incisor (I^3, 103) in Fig. 2-19.

Wry bite

A wry bite is a condition in which the central incisors of the mandible and maxilla do not align evenly. It may be caused by uneven mandibular lengths or by the failure of

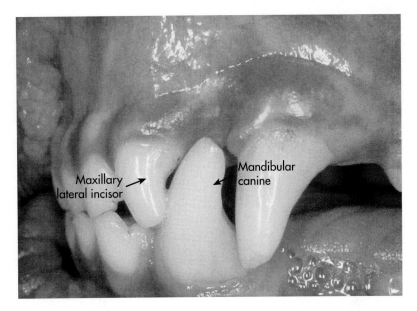

FIGURE 2-18 Maxillary lateral incisor occluding against the mandibular canine.

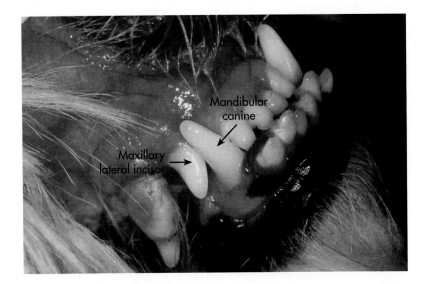

FIGURE 2-19 Mandibular canine occluding labial to the maxillary lateral incisor.

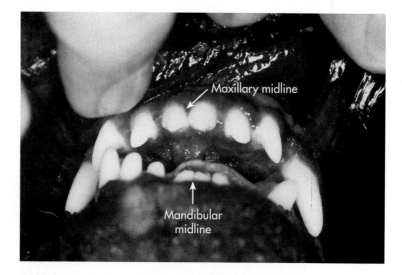

FIGURE 2-20 The mandibular and maxillary central incisors do not align.

the maxilla to develop evenly. The origin of wry bite may be genetic (inheritance of uneven jaw lengths), or the condition may be caused by trauma to the bones during development of the facial structure. Treatment ranges from extraction of teeth to placement of orthodontic appliances. The symbol is "WRY." Note that in Fig. 2-20 the central incisors do not align. The right mandibular canine (C_1, 404) is occluding mesial-labial to the right lateral maxillary incisor (I^3, 103).

Iatrogenic orthodontic disease

Occasionally, clients (or even veterinarians and office staff) make misguided attempts to correct orthodontic problems. These efforts may cause severe malalignments of teeth. In Fig. 2-21 an elastic has been placed around the mandibular canine ($_1C_1$, 304, 404) and incisors ($_{321}I_{123}$, 301, 302, 303, 401, 402, 403). The result is severe displacement of the incisors and canines toward the center of the mouth.

Periodontal Disease

Gingivitis

Gingivitis is inflammation of the gingiva. Most often, it is caused by bacterial plaque. A number of conditions should be indicated in the chart of a patient with periodontal disease; these conditions will be discussed in the chapters on prophylaxis and periodontal therapy. Fig. 2-22 shows a moderate amount of plaque and calculus on the left maxillary third (^3P, 207) and fourth premolars (^4P, 208). Gingival inflammation is minimal, however, and the patient is expected to respond positively to professional hygiene and home care.

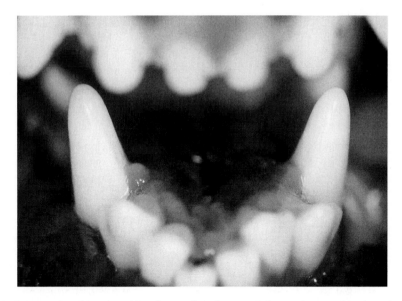

FIGURE 2-21 A rubber band has been placed around the canines and incisors in an unsuccessful attempt to move the mandibular incisors lingually.

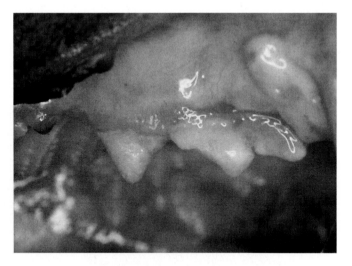

FIGURE 2-22 Gingivitis in a cat.

Periodontitis

Periodontitis affects the surrounding tissues of the tooth. This condition is the most common oral disease among dogs and cats. The staging, treatment, and prevention of periodontal disease are discussed in Chapters 7 and 9.

Feline Stomatitis and Faucitis

Feline stomatitis, or faucitis, syndrome is a devastating condition. Cats with this syndrome typically have extremely red and inflamed tissues in the oral cavity. The oral cavity is typically described as having a cobblestone appearance (see Chapter 13). Severe inflammation at the commissures that extends into the fauca is visible in Fig. 2-23.

Adverse Conditions of the Tooth Surface

Stains

Stains result from occlusal wear and exposure of dentine. They are not necessarily pathologic, although many clients ask for a consultation when they think caries are present. *[Caries. A demineralization and loss of tooth structure resulting from the action of microorganisms on carbohydrates.]* Enamel normally resists staining, whereas dentine is porous and stains easily. In Fig. 2-24 the left maxillary first molar (^{1}M, 209) shows wear and a dark dentinal stain. The white material in the occlusal pit is food particles.

Abrasions

Abrasions result from the repeated friction of the teeth against an external object, such as hair or toys. One common cause of wear is the chewing (and spinning or

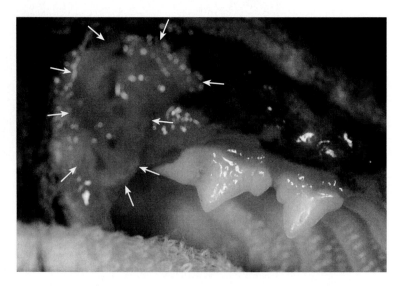

FIGURE 2-23 Severe inflammation of the fauca *(arrows)*.

rolling in the mouth) of tennis balls. Trapped dirt in the fibers covering the tennis ball creates a sandpaper-like surface. The symbol for abrasion is "AB." The patient in Fig. 2-25 suffers from chronic skin disease and chews its hair as a result. Its mandibular incisors ($_{321}I_{123}$, 301, 302, 303, 401, 402, 403) and canines ($_1C_1$, 304, 404) show severe wear.

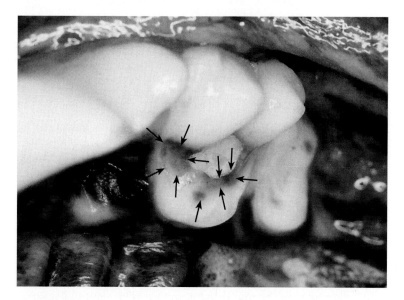

FIGURE 2-24 Dentinal stain *(arrows)* on the maxillary left first molar.

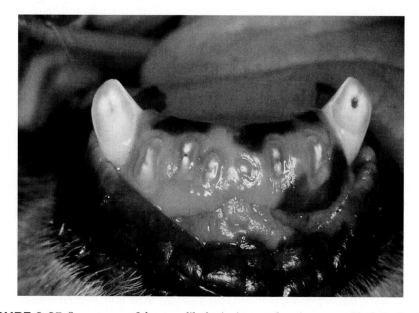

FIGURE 2-25 Severe wear of the mandibular incisors and canines caused by hair chewing.

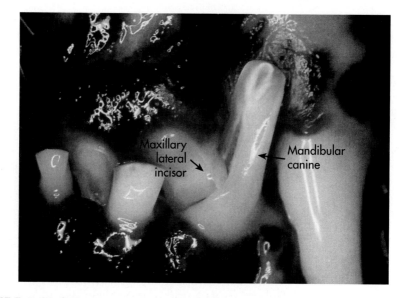

FIGURE 2-26 Severe wear caused by malocclusion. Note the maxillary lateral incisor grooved into the mandibular canine.

Attrition

Attrition results from the friction of teeth against each other. Fig. 2-26 shows severe wear of the mandibular canine. The symbol for attrition is "AT." The patient in Fig. 2-26 may have had an occlusion similar to that shown in Fig. 2-18 (Class III occlusion, mandibular prognathism). The mandibular left canine ($_1$C, 304) shows severe wear resulting from friction against the left maxillary lateral incisor (C, 203).

Enamel hypoplasia

Cells called *ameloblasts* create enamel. If these cells are debilitated, they stop producing enamel. The area of the crown no longer has a shiny surface; instead, it is dull and susceptible to flaking. This condition is called *enamel hypoplasia*. Conditions that cause a temporary debilitation of the patient, such as high fever, may cause enamel hypoplasia. Trauma or traumatic extractions of primary teeth may also be causes. The symbol for enamel hypoplasia is "EH." An injury such as that shown on the right mandibular canine (C_1, 404) in Fig. 2-27 may have resulted from an infection similar to the one that caused the fractured tooth in Fig. 2-7. Note also that the patient in Fig. 2-27 has a severely retrusive mandible.

Caries

Caries (also called *cavities*) occur in dogs and cats. The most common types are Class I caries, which are pits and fissures on the occlusal surfaces of teeth, and Class V caries, which occur on the buccal and labial surfaces. Treatment options depend on the depth of the lesion and include extraction, simple restorations, endodontic therapy, and crown restorations.

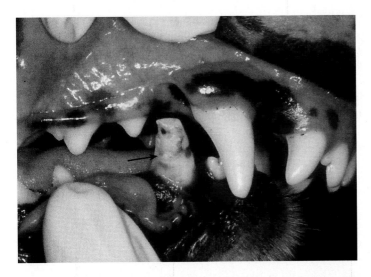

FIGURE 2-27 Enamel hypoplasia in a dog with a severely retrusive mandible.

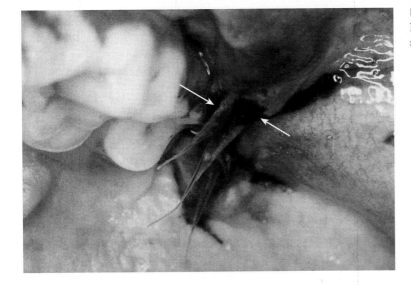

FIGURE 2-28 Foxtail awns lodged behind the maxillary second molar.

Class V caries occur on the gingival third of the crown of the tooth, on the buccal or lingual surface. These are common in cats and are discussed (and classified) in Chapter 13.

Foreign Bodies

Foreign bodies are sometimes caught on the tooth or trapped in the oral cavity. Rubber bands may be wrapped around teeth, and bones may become lodged between teeth. The retention of this foreign material can cause infection and even tooth loss. The patient in Fig. 2-28 had foxtail weed awns lodged behind the left maxillary second molar ([2]M, 210).

Endodontic Disease

Endodontics is the treatment of diseases inside the tooth. Endodontic disease may be caused by fractures, trauma, and iatrogenic *[Iatrogenic. A condition caused by the health-care provider]* factors, such as overheating the tooth during cleaning procedures.

Fracture classification

Collisions with automobiles and the catching or chewing of hard objects are common causes of fractures. Numerous fracture classification schemes, patterned after those used in human dentistry, exist in veterinary dentistry. For the most part, these classes do not apply to veterinary dentistry. The fracture classification system described in this text simplifies the fracture to the depth of fracture (e.g., enamel only, dentine only, pulp, subgingival).

Class 1

A Class 1 fracture is a chip fracture that has caused only the loss of enamel. Many of these Class 1 fractures are insignificant and do not require treatment. The fracture is charted by the symbols "FX1" and a jagged line over the area of the fracture.

Class 2

A Class 2 fracture involves both enamel and dentine but has not entered the pulp chamber. *[Pulp. Soft tissue component of the tooth consisting of blood, vascular tissue, nerve tissue, loose connective tissue, and cellular elements such as odontoblasts that form dentine.]* Patients with Class 2 fractures may not require treatment, depending on the depth of the fracture and age of the patient. The fracture is charted by the symbols "FX2" and a jagged line over the area of the fracture. In Fig. 2-29 the patient has a Class 2 fracture of the left mandibular canine ($_1$C, 304) that involves enamel and dentine but has not entered the pulp, nor has any part of the tooth been fractured below the gumline.

Class 2b

In a Class 2b fracture, enamel and dentine are involved and the pulp chamber is not exposed, although the fracture extends below the gumline. This type of fracture may require no treatment, endodontic or periodontic treatment, or both. The fracture is charted by the symbols "FX2b" and a jagged line over the area of the fracture.

Class 3

A Class 3 fracture penetrates the enamel and dentine and exposes the pulp chamber. This type of fracture requires extraction or endodontic therapy. The fracture is charted by the symbols "FX3" and a jagged line over the area of the fracture. Fig. 2-30 shows a fractured or worn right maxillary canine (C^1, 104) with pulp exposure. These fractures also occur in cats. The left maxillary canine (^{1}C, 204) in Fig. 2-31 has an acute fracture, as demonstrated by the hemorrhage over the crown.

Class 3b

A Class 3b fracture involves enamel and dentine, exposes the pulp chamber, and extends below the gumline. This type of fracture requires extraction or endodontic

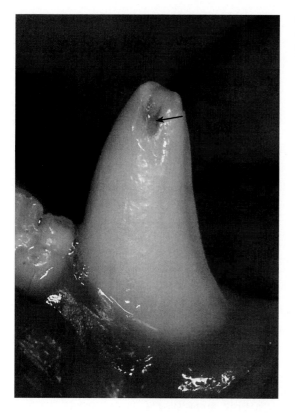

FIGURE 2-29 Fracture *(arrow)* of the enamel that extends partly into the dentine but not into the pulp.

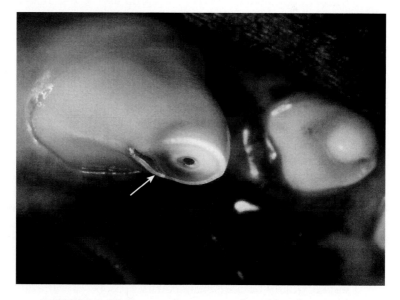

FIGURE 2-30 Fractured or worn canine with pulp exposure.

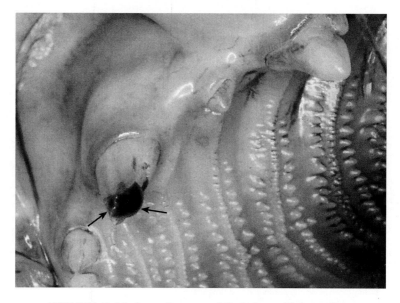

FIGURE 2-31 Acute fracture of the left maxillary canine.

therapy and possible periodontal treatment. The fracture is charted by the symbols "FX3b" and a jagged line over the area of the fracture. Fig. 2-32 shows a fractured right maxillary fourth premolar (P4, 108); because of the depth of the fracture and the periodontal involvement, extraction may be the treatment of choice.

Class 4
A Class 4 fracture involves the root. The tooth is often quite mobile and, depending on the location, may require extraction. The fracture is charted by the symbols "FX4" and a jagged line over the area of the fracture. This radiograph shows a fracture of the left mandibular central incisor (₁I, 301). Treatment for the tooth shown in Fig. 2-33 is extraction.

Fractures of specific tooth types
Incisors
Incisors can fracture or deteriorate with wear. Fractures of the incisors often result from running into hard objects; catching baseballs, golf balls, and rocks; fighting; and chewing enclosures to escape. Wear occurs most commonly by chewing skin. The friction of teeth against teeth associated with malocclusion also results in wear, as does the chewing of rocks, bones, and other hard objects. Patients who chronically chew certain toys, such as tennis balls and cloth Frisbees, may also wear down their teeth. Practitioners sometimes overlook disease of the mandibular incisors in awake patients because the maxillary incisors cover the labial side when the mouth

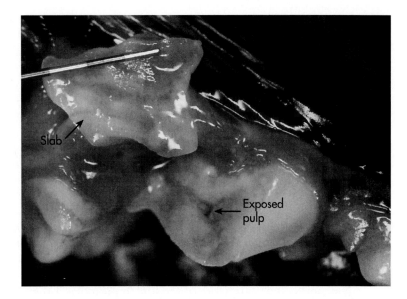

FIGURE 2-32 Fractured fourth premolar with the slab still attached and the pulp chamber exposed.

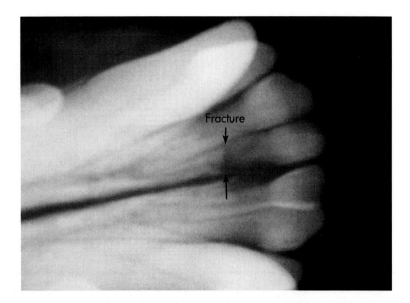

FIGURE 2-33 Root fracture requiring extraction of the tooth and root fragment.

is closed and the tongue covers the lingual side when the mouth is open. Fractures of the maxillary incisors may be difficult to see because they often occur on the palatal side. Fig. 2-34 shows severe wear of the mandibular canines ($_1C_1$, 304, 404) and incisors ($_{321}I_{123}$, 301, 302, 303, 401, 402, 403).

Canines
The canines are susceptible to trauma because they are the most exposed teeth, located in the front of the oral cavity, and they have long crowns. The canines have several important functions. In addition to their holding and tearing functions, the mandibular canines may act as a guide for the tongue. The maxillary canines serve to hold the lip out and away from the gums. Without these teeth, many patients pinch or bite their lips between the mandibular canines and gums. Like the incisors, canines are fractured when patients fight and chew, catch, and run into hard objects. Wear occurs by excessive or inappropriate chewing and occlusion abnormalities. The patient in Fig. 2-35, a tennis-ball chewer, exhibits table wear on the crowns of all visible teeth.

Premolars
The most common fracture of the fourth premolar is the "slab" fracture. This fracture results from the force that is placed on a very small area of tooth (cusp) when the patient bites down. The shear force fractures enamel and dentine, exposing the pulp. For this reason the chewing of hard objects, such as hooves, bones, pig's ears, and pressed rawhide products, is discouraged. In Fig. 2-36 the cusp of the right maxillary fourth premolar (P^4, 108) has been compressed into the pulp chamber, moving a slab buccally.

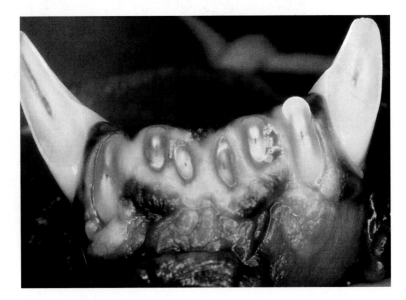

FIGURE 2-34 Severe wear of the canines and incisors.

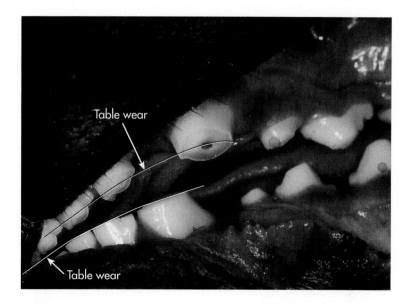

FIGURE 2-35 Table wear (lines) on teeth caused by chewing on a tennis ball.

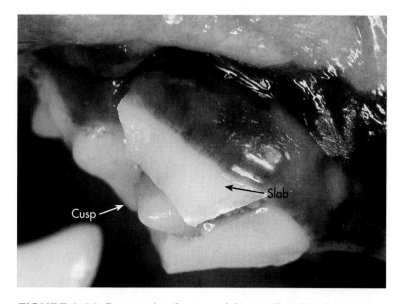

FIGURE 2-36 Compression fracture of the maxillary fourth premolar.

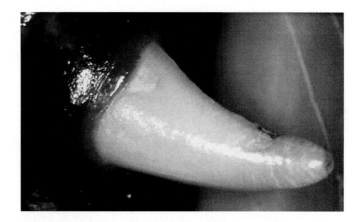

FIGURE 2-37 Traumatic injury has caused pulpal hemorrhage, resulting in a purple discoloration of the canine.

Molars

Fractures of the molars usually occur in combination with fractures of the maxillary fourth premolar. When patients chew extremely hard objects, the same forces are applied to the mandibular first molar as to the maxillary fourth premolar. Practitioners may miss these fractures during physical exams because the tongue overlaps the teeth when the mouth is open and the maxillary fourth premolars and molars cover them when the mouth is closed.

Tooth discoloration

The teeth and cusps take on a variety of colors that may indicate a pathologic condition. The normal, healthy tooth is white. If wear has exposed dentine, the exposed portion appears brown. If the pulp has been exposed, it appears black and the tooth loses its translucent appearance. Pink, purple, or tan teeth indicate pulpal hemorrhage.

Purple discoloration indicates pulpal hemorrhage. The most common cause of hemorrhage is trauma to the tooth. This trauma may result from being hit by a car, running into a solid object, or colliding with another dog's tooth. Trauma may lead to pulpitis, which is a pulpal inflammation that may be reversible. If it is irreversible, the pulp hemorrhages and dies as a result of the increased internal pressure in the tooth, which causes crushing and death of cells. The odontoblasts that line the pulp chamber and guard the dentinal tubules also die, which allows blood cells to enter the tooth. At first, the result is a pink tooth. As the hemoglobin loses oxygen, the tooth changes to purple and later to tan. The left maxillary canine ([1]C, 204) shown in Fig. 2-37 is purple. The recommended treatment for this tooth is root canal therapy.

Luxations

Luxation is partial displacement of the tooth from the socket. In Fig. 2-38 the left maxillary canine ([1]C, 204) has rotated at the apex. The tooth may still be vital. Immediate repositioning and splinting is recommended. Root canal therapy may be necessary.

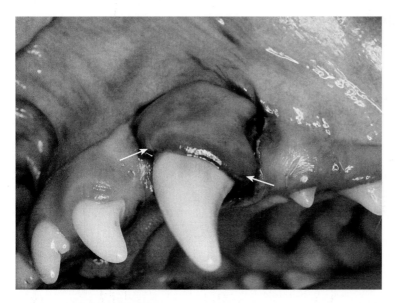

FIGURE 2-38 Luxated left maxillary canine caused by a dogfight.

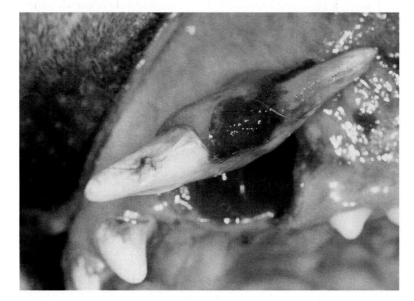

FIGURE 2-39 Avulsion of the maxillary canine.

Avulsions

Avulsion is complete displacement of the tooth from the socket. If the tooth is to be saved, it must be replaced immediately. Special solutions are available to help preserve the lost tooth, but usually they are not readily available. Clients may place the tooth in milk as a first aid measure. Endodontic therapy is required (see Chapter 12). In Fig. 2-39 the left maxillary canine ([1]C, 204) has been avulsed from the socket. Saving this tooth requires immediate replacement and splinting followed by root canal therapy 6 weeks later.

Electrical cord shock

Tooth damage caused by chewing electrical cords may not be discovered for days or even months after the injury. If the injury occurs when the patient is very young, severe damage may occur and the affected teeth may require extraction. The maxillary fourth premolar or first molar and the mandibular first molar are usually involved. The patient in Fig. 2-40 received an electrical shock at a very early age, as evidenced by the pulp chamber of the left mandibular first molar ($_1$M, 309), which is large and undeveloped compared with the pulp chambers of adjacent teeth.

Odontoclastic Resorptive Lesions

The cause, or causes, of feline odontoclastic resorptive lesion syndrome (FORL) is not known. These lesions were first discovered at the neck of the tooth, the area where the root and crown come together. They were therefore first known as "neck lesions." These lesions have since been given a number of other names: *resorptive lesions, cervical line lesions,* and *feline cavities.* The tooth resorbs and is eventually lost. Staging and treatment of this disease are discussed in Chapter 13.

Oral Medical Disease

Oronasal fistulas

Oronasal fistulas result from advanced periodontal disease on the inside of the canines. As the plate of bone between the canine and the nasal cavity breaks down, fistulas develop. They are often present but not diagnosed before the extraction of the canine. Oronasal fistulas are documented by indicating the missing tooth and noting "ONF"

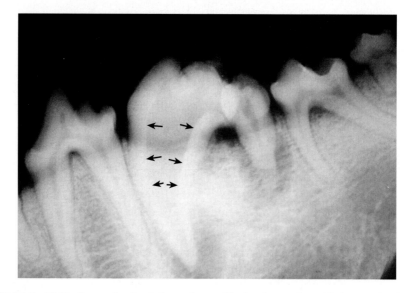

FIGURE 2-40 Radiograph of a deformed mandibular first molar with incompletely developed pulp chamber *(arrows).* Trauma was caused by an electrical cord shock.

in the chart. The patient in Fig. 2-41 has lost its right maxillary canine (C^1, 104) as a result of chronic periodontal disease. A hole exists that opens to the nasal cavity.

Uremic ulceration

Patients with advanced renal disease may develop ulcerations on the tip of the tongue. Increased calculus formation and periodontal disease are associated problems—all the more reason that preoperative blood profiles should be run before oral procedures are performed. Fig. 2-42 shows ulcerations along the tongue margins that were caused by uremia.

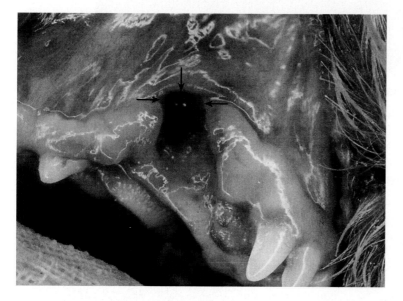

FIGURE 2-41 Oronasal fistula *(arrows)* of the right maxillary canine.

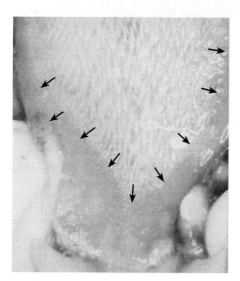

FIGURE 2-42 Ulcerations *(arrows)* of the margins of the tongue caused by uremia (the BUN was greater than 250).

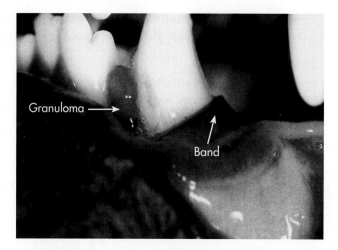

FIGURE 2-43 Granuloma caused by a rubber band around the mandibular canine.

Oral Neoplasia

Benign tumors

While they may grow locally and in rare instances convert to malignant tumors, benign tumors generally do not spread deep into tissue or metastasize to lymph nodes or lungs. Benign tumors respond well to surgical removal. If not completely removed, however, they may return to the same or an adjacent location.

Granulomas

Benign granulomas are common and usually result from periodontal disease or other irritation. They respond well to local excision and removal of the originating cause (Fig. 2-43).

Gingival hyperplasia

Gingival hyperplasia, the proliferation of gingival cells, is common among some breeds, particularly the collie, boxer, and cocker spaniel. Pocket formation and periodontal disease may result from this hyperplastic tissue. Fig. 2-44 shows gingival hyperplasia of the left maxillary canine ([1]C, 204) and first premolar ([1]P, 205), which is completely covered.

Fibromatous epulis

Fibromatous epulides are characterized by the presence of a tumor in the tissues of the gingiva. A fibromatous epulis contains primarily fibrous tissues. Generally, the fibromatous epulis responds well to excision; however, it may return if the excision is incomplete. The symbol is "EP."

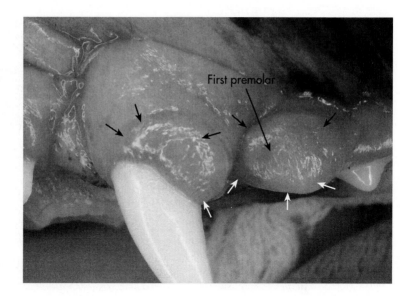

First premolar

FIGURE 2-44 Gingival hyperplasia around the maxillary canine, which completely covers the first premolar.

Ossifying epulis

An ossifying epulis resembles a fibromatous epulis but also contains large amounts of bone material, which give it a bony quality apparent during excision. Because of the depth of the bone, these tumors sometimes are difficult to remove.

Malignant tumors
Acanthomatous epulis

The acanthomatous epulis is primarily composed of epithelial cells associated with the tissue. These epulides tend to invade bone, which makes dental radiographic evaluation important. Most of the time, acanthomatous epulides are located in the rostral portion of the oral cavity. This is not always the case, however, as shown by the tumor located around the left mandibular fourth premolar ($_4$P, 308) and first molar ($_1$M, 309) in Fig. 2-45.

Malignant melanoma

Malignant melanomas occur on any site in the oral cavity: gingiva, buccal mucosa, hard and soft palates, and tongue. They are locally invasive and highly metastatic to the lungs, regional lymph nodes, and bone. As with many malignancies, clients may first notice a minor change, such as bad breath. Clients also sometimes report oral bleeding. Malignant tumors may appear darkly pigmented or nonpigmented. Loose teeth, caused by bone involvement, is another symptom. The prognosis is poor because reoccurrence is common. Fig. 2-46 shows a malignant melanoma of the maxilla.

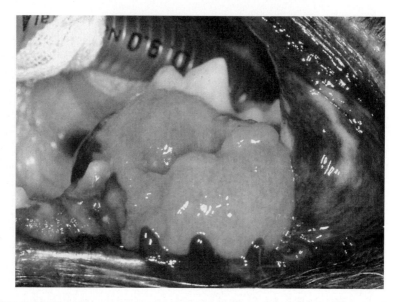

FIGURE 2-45 Usually present in the anterior portion of the mouth, this acanthomatous epulis is located around the fourth premolar and first molar.

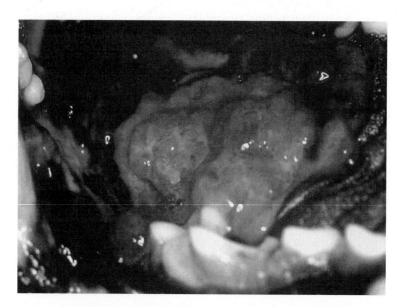

FIGURE 2-46 Malignant melanoma of the maxilla.

Fibrosarcoma

Fibrosarcomas occur in the mandible or maxilla. They may create fleshy, protruding, firm masses that sometimes are friable. As the masses grow, they can become ulcerated and infected. Most of the time, it is the local growth that becomes the problem rather than the spreading of this tumor to the lymph nodes or lungs.

Squamous cell carcinoma

Squamous cell carcinomas arise in a variety of locations in the mouth. Their cell type is from the epithelium. They can occur in tonsillar crypts and the gingiva. Their appearance varies, but generally they are nodular, grey to pink, irregular masses that invade the bone and cause tooth mobility. Generally, the farther away from tonsils or the floor of the mouth, the better the prognosis. Fig. 2-47 shows squamous cell carcinoma of the right tonsil of a cat. The prognosis is poor.

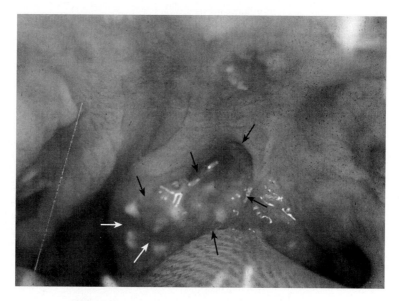

FIGURE 2-47 Tonsillar squamous cell carcinoma.

LIST OF DIAGNOSTIC CODES (ADAPTED FROM THE AVDC TRACKING COMMITTEE RECOMMENDATIONS)*

2D	Secondary dentine	C8	Root apex
AB	Abrasion	CA	Cavity—fracture or defect (1-8)
AL	Attachment loss		
APG	Apexigenesis	CAL	Calculus
APX	Apexification	CC	Curettage closed
AT	Attrition	CFL	Cleft lip
AXB	Anterior cross-bite	CFP	Cleft palate
BF	Broken file	CI	Calculus index
BG	Buccal granuloma	CMO	Craniomandibular osteodystrophy
BL	Bone recession		
BSF	Broken spiral filler	CO	Curettage open
C/MOD	Cavity—mesial occlusal distal surface	CON	Consultation
		CU	Contact ulcer ("kissing" ulcer)
C1	Occlusal or pit and fissure; molars and premolars		
		CWD	Crowding
C1N	Class 1	DB	Dentinal bonding agent
C1O	Class 1 occlusion: normal with one or more teeth out of alignment or rotated	DC	Dentigerous cyst
		DR	Dilacerated root
		DT/D	Deciduous tooth
		ED	Enamel defect
C1V	Class 1	EG	Eosinophilic granuloma
C2	MOD: Mesioocclusodistal, mesiooclusal, occluso-distal, molars and premolars	EGC	EG lip/cheilitis (lip)
		EGL	EG lingual/tongue
		EH	Enamel hypocalcification/hypoplasia
C2O	Class 2 occlusion: brachygnathism; overshot; retrusive mandible; distal mandibular excursion	EP	Epulis fibromatous
		EX	Excision
		EXT	Extrusion
		FB	Foreign body
		FE	Furcation exposure
C3	Mesial or distal; incisor no ridge	FE1	Furcation exposure, Class 1: (probe can barely detect the entrance to the furcation)
C3O	Class 3 occlusion: prognathism; undershot; protrusive mandible; mesial mandibular excursion		
		FE2	Furcation exposure, Class 2: (probe can enter furcation but cannot reach other side)
C4	Mesioincisodistal, mesio-incisal, incisodistal, incisor with ridge		
		FE3	Furcation exposure, Class 3: (probe can pass through furcation to the other side)
C5	Lingual or facial		
C6	Cusp		
C7	Root	FEN	Fenestration

*Wiggs RB, Lobprise HP: *Veterinary dentistry: principles and practice,* Philadelphia, 1997, Lippincott-Raven; Holmstrom SE, Frost P, Eisner ER: *Veterinary dental techniques,* Philadelphia, 1998, WB Saunders.

FRE	Frenectomy	OW	Occlusal wear
FRN	Frenotomy	P&F	Pit and fissure
FX	Fracture	P3	Periodontal pocket 3 mm
GCF	Gingival crevicular fluid	P4	Periodontal pocket 4 mm
GH	Gingival hyperplasia/ hypertrophy	P5	Periodontal pocket 5 mm
		P6	Periodontal pocket 6 mm
GI	Gingivitis index (Loe and Silness)	P7	Periodontal pocket 7 mm
		P8	Periodontal pocket 8 mm
GI0	Gingivitis index, Grade 0: normal gingivitis	P9	Periodontal pocket 9 mm
		PAP	Papillomatosis
GI1	Gingivitis index , Grade 1: mild inflammation	PD	Palatal defect
		PD1	Periodontal disease, Stage 1: initial stage
GI2	Gingivitis index, Grade 2: moderate inflammation	PD2	Periodontal disease, Stage 2: early stage
GI3	Gingivitis index, Grade 3: severe inflammation	PD3	Periodontal disease, Stage 3: established stage
GLS	Glossitis	PD4	Periodontal disease, Stage 4: advanced stage
GM	Gingival margin		
GP	Gutta percha	PDI	Periodontal disease index
GR	Gingival recession	PDL	Periodontal ligament
HT	Hairy tongue	PE	Pulp exposure
INT	Intrusion	PEM	Pemphigus
KL	Kissing lesion	PERF	Perforation
LFD	Lip fold dermatitis	PG	Periodontal pocket gingival (pseudopocket)
LG	Lingual granuloma		
LPS	Lymphocytic plasmacytic stomatitis	PI	Plaque index (Silness and Loe)
LUP	Lupus erythematosus	PI0	Plaque index, Grade 0: no plaque
M0	Mobility: normal or none		
M1	Mobility: slight	PI1	Plaque index, Grade 1: thin film of plaque at gingival margin visible when checked with explorer
M2	Mobility: moderate		
M3	Mobility: severe		
MAL	Malocclusion (modified angle classification)		
MAL1	Cross-bite	PI2	Plaque index, Grade 2: moderate amount of plaque along gingival margin; interdental space free of plaque; plaque visible
MAL2	Brachygnathia		
MAL3	Prognathia		
MGL	Mucogingival loss		
MGM	Mucogingival margin		
MM	Mucous membrane		
MN/FX	Mandible fracture	PI3	Plaque index, Grade 3: heavy plaque accumulation at gingival margin; interdental space filled with plaque
MX/FX	Maxillary fracture		
NE	Near exposure		
NV	Nonvital		
O	Circle around missing tooth on chart		
		PIB	Periodontal pocket infrabony
OAF	Oroantral fistula		
OM	Oral mass	PLQ	Plaque
ONF	Oronasal fistula	PLT	Palate
OST	Osteomyelitis		

PP	Periodontal pocket	SYM/S	Symphysis separation
PSB	Periodontal pocket suprabony	SZ	Zygomatic salivary gland
		TA	Tooth avulsed
PT	Palatal trauma defect	TIP	Tipping
PT/P	Permanent tooth	TL	Tooth luxated
PXB	Posterior cross-bite	TMJ/DL	Temporomandibular joint dislocation
RD	Retained deciduous tooth		
RE	Root exposure	TMJ/DP	Temporomandibular joint dysplasia
RL	Resorptive lesion (FORL: feline odontoclastic resorptive lesion)	TMJ/FX	Temporomandibular joint fracture
		TMJ/L	Temporomandibular joint luxation
ROT	Rotation		
RR	Retained root	TRANS	Body movement or translation
RTR	Retained root		
SAL	Salivary gland	VBL/NV	Vital/nonvital bleaching
SBI	Sulcus bleeding index	VT	Vital tooth
SE	Staining extrinsic (metal)	W1	Periodontal bony pocket 1 wall
SER	Supereruption		
SI	Staining intrinsic (blood)	W2	Periodontal bony pocket 2 wall
SL	Sublingual		
SLG	Sublingual granuloma	W3	Periodontal bony pocket 3 wall
SM	Mandibular salivary gland		
SN	Supernumerary	W4/CUP	Periodontal bony pocket 4 wall cup lesion
SP	Parotid salivary gland		
SS	Sublingual salivary gland	WRY	Wry mouth
STM	Stomatitis	XRFM	X-ray full mouth
SUL	Sulcus	ZOE	Zinc oxide eugenol
SYM	Symphysis		

LIST OF TREATMENT CODES (AS ADAPTED FROM THE AVDC TRACKING COMMITTEE RECOMMENDATIONS.)*

ACY	Acrylic	CAM	Crown amputation reduction
AP	Alveoloplasty		
AS	Apical sealer/cement	CBU	Core build-up
BE	Biopsy excisional	CFP/R	Cleft palate repair
BFR	Buccal fold removal	CFW	Circumferential wiring
BG	Bone graft	CM	Crown-metal (CMG=gold CMB=base metal, etc.)
BI	Biopsy incisional		
BKT	Bracket	CON	Consultation
BP	Bridge pontic	CR	Crown
BR	Bridge	CS	Culture/sensitivity
BRC	Bridge cantilever	CT	Citric acid treatment
BRM	Bridge Maryland	CUL	Culture

*Wiggs RB, Lobprise HB: *Veterinary dentistry: principles and practice,* Philadelphia, 1997, Lippincott-Raven; Holmstrom SE, Frost P, Eisner ER: *Veterinary dental techniques,* Philadelphia, 1998, WB Saunders.

EC	Elastic chain (power chain)	P&FS	Pit and fissure sealer
EX	Excision	PC	Pulp capping
FAR	Flap apically repositioning	PCD	Direct pulp capping
FCR	Flap coronally repositioning	PCI	Indirect pulp capping
FG	Fluoride gel	PFM	Crown—porcelain fused to
FGG	Flap free gingival graft		metal
FLS	Flap lateral sliding	PRO	Prophylaxis complete
FR-P/P	Fracture repair pin/plate/	PS	Periodontal surgery
	splint/screw (SC)/wire (W)	R	Restoration
FRB	Flap reverse bevel	R/A	Restoration amalgam
FV	Fluoride varnish	R/C	Restoration composite
GP	Gingivoplasty	R/I	Restoration glass ionomer
GTR	Guided tissue regeneration	RCS	Surgical root canal
GV	Gingivectomy	RCT	Root canal therapy
HS	Hemisection	RGF	Retrograde filling (RGF/A
IDW	Interdental wiring		= amalgam, etc.)
IL	Inlay	RP	Root planing
IM	Impressions/models (ortho-	RPC	Closed root planing
	dontic or restorative)	RPO	Open root planing
IMP	Implant	RRX	Root resection (hemisection)
IO	Interceptive orthodontics	SC	Subgingival curettage
IOD	Interceptive orthodontics	SM	Surgery—mandibulectomy
	deciduous tooth	SO	Surgical orthopedics
IOP	Interceptive orthodontics	SP	Surgery—palate
	permanent tooth	SPF	Scale polish fluoride
OA	Orthodontic appliance	SPL	Splint
OAA	Orthodontic appliance—	SX	Surgery—maxillectomy
	adjust	T	Bracket marked on chart
OAI	Ortho appliance—install	TP	Treatment plan
OAR	Ortho appliance—remove	TRX	Tooth resection
OC	Orthodontic consultation		(hemisection)
	(genetic counseling)	VER	Veneer
OI	Osseous implant	VP	Vital pulpotomy
OL	Onlay	WIR	Wire
ONF/R	Oronasal fistula repair or	X	Simple extraction
	restore	XR	X-ray
OP	Odontoplasty	XS	Extraction with sectioning
OR	Orthodontic recheck		of tooth
OSW	Osseous wiring	XSS	Surgical extraction

Worksheet

STUDENT NAME:_____

1. The primary teeth are also known as _____ or _____ teeth.

2. _____ orthodontics is the process of extracting primary teeth when it appears that they will cause orthodontic malocclusions.

3. Cranial mandibular osteodystrophy occurs in primarily _____ _____ _____ _____.

4. A Class _____ occlusion is said to occur when the mandible is shorter than normal.

5. The condition known as *maxillary brachygnathism* is caused by a _____ maxilla.

6. A _____ bite is a condition in which the central incisors of the mandible and the maxilla do not align evenly.

7. _____ is inflammation of the gingiva.

8. _____ disease is disease of the surrounding tissues of the tooth.

9. _____ normally resists staining, whereas _____ is porous and stains easily.

10. _____ result from the friction of teeth against an external object, such as hair or a tennis ball.

11. _____ occurs as the result of the friction of teeth against each other.

12. _____ _____ can result from conditions that cause a temporary debilitation of the patient, such as high fever.

13. _____ is the treatment of diseases inside the tooth.

14. A fracture that has penetrated enamel and dentine and involved the pulp chamber should be treated by _____ or _____.

15. The most common fracture of the fourth premolar is the _____ fracture.

16. Purple discoloration indicates _____ in the pulp.

17. An _____ is the displacement of the tooth from the socket.

18. Feline odontoclastic resorptive lesion syndrome is also known as "_____ _____ _____."

19. _____ tumors generally do not spread deep into tissue or metastasize to lymph node or lungs.

20. As with many oral malignancies, clients may first notice a minor change, such as _____ _____.

3

Dental Instruments and Equipment

Veterinary dentistry is a very instrument- and equipment-intensive profession. An ample assortment of seemingly similar instruments are required for the proper performance of dental procedures. This chapter is devoted to the instruments and equipment required for the prevention and treatment of periodontal disease. The equipment and materials required for dental radiology and other procedures are discussed in subsequent chapters.

ORGANIZATION OF THE DENTAL DEPARTMENT

For the successful treatment of patients, veterinary dentistry requires many instruments and materials. The great number of tools necessitates sufficient shelf space and a practical method for keeping track of each item. A card file or a book with photographs identifying each item's proper place is important for organization.

HAND INSTRUMENTS

Veterinary technicians and practitioners use four main types of hand instruments (Fig. 3-1). Most instruments have four specific parts: handle, shank, terminal shank, and working end. Handles, the parts that are grasped, come in a variety of round, tapered, and hexagonal shapes. The best handle shape for the procedure depends on individual preference. The shank joins the working end with the handle. The length and curvature of the shank determines the teeth that the instrument will be able to access. The terminal shank is the part of the shank that is closest to the working end. The working end of the instrument is the portion that comes in contact with the tooth.

Explorers

Although explorers and periodontal probes are actually two different types of instruments, they are grouped together because they are usually manufactured as

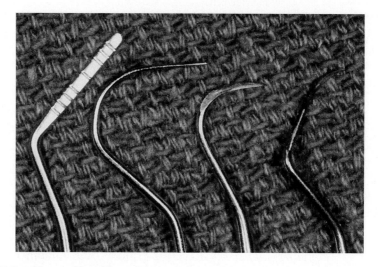

FIGURE 3-1 Types of hand instruments *(left to right)*: probe, explorer, scaler, curette. Each type of instrument is available in a variety of styles.

double-ended instruments. One end is the periodontal probe, and the other end the explorer. Explorers are used to detect plaque and calculus. They are also used to explore for cavities and check for exposed pulp chambers. The design of the explorer increases the operator's tactile sensitivity. There are a variety of color banded probes available. Some have bands at 2 mm, others at 3 mm and others a combination of 2 mm and 3 mm.

Shepherd's hook

The shepherd's hook (or crook) is the most commonly found explorer. These instruments are manufactured in combination with the periodontal probe (Fig. 3-2).

Pigtail explorer

The curved shape of the pigtail explorer allows the operator to use the tip of the instrument and thereby avoid touching with the side of the instruments those parts of the tooth that are not being explored (Fig. 3-3). Pigtail explorers usually come hooked to the right on one end and to the left on the other, allowing for a greater range of exploration. The explorer functions by gliding along the tooth surface in search of irregularities and magnifies the user's tactile sense.

Periodontal Probes

Many styles of periodontal probes are available (Fig. 3-4). The probe on the far left of Fig. 3-4 features color bands every 3 mm. There are six bands, which means that this probe is capable of measuring 18 mm. The probe on the middle left is notched. It has major bands every 5 mm, with three intermediate bands every 1 mm. The 4-, 9-, and 14-mm small bands are skipped. This probe is capable of measuring 15 mm.

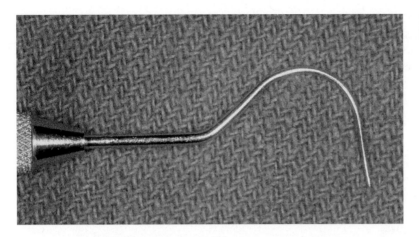

FIGURE 3-2 Shepherd's hook explorer.

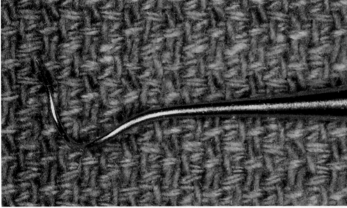

FIGURE 3-3 Pigtail explorer.

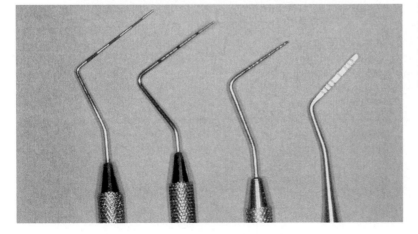
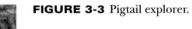

FIGURE 3-4 Four types of periodontal probes *(left to right)*: Cislak 18-mm periodontal probe, Hu-Friedy 15-mm probe, notched round probe, and flat notched probe.

The middle right probe is the traditional 1-cm type. It has the following notch formula: notch at 1, 2, and 3 mm; 4 mm skipped; notch at 5 mm; 6 mm skipped; notch at 7, 8, 9, and 10 mm. The probe on the far right is a flat probe. To use the periodontal probe, the technician or practitioner gently inserts the probe into the pocket or sulcus to evaluate its depth.

Calculus Removal Forceps

The calculus removal forceps allow for quick removal of large pieces of calculus (Fig. 3-5). The instrument has tips of different lengths and shapes. The longer tip is placed over the crown, and the shorter tip is placed under the calculus. Calculus is sheared off the tooth when the two parts of the handle are brought together. When using this instrument, the technician or practitioner must be careful not to damage the enamel surface or gingiva.

Scalers

Scalers have three sharp sides and a sharp tip. These instruments are used for scaling calculus from the crown surface. They are particularly useful in removing calculus from narrow but deep fissures, such as that located on the buccal surface of the fourth premolar. Scalers are used for supragingival scaling only. Because they may damage the gingiva and periodontal ligament, scalers should not be used subgingivally. The ends of the instrument are usually mirror images of each other, which allows adaptation to opposite surfaces.

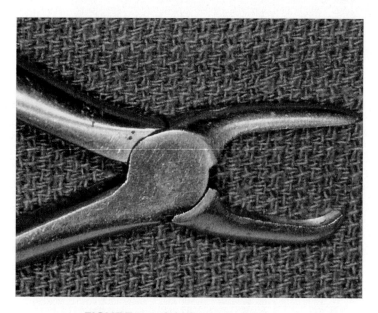

FIGURE 3-5 Calculus removal forceps.

Scalers have a sharp point, or a tip (T). The face (F) is the flat side of the instrument between the two cutting edges. The cutting edge (C), the working portion of the scaler, is the confluence of the face and the sides (Fig. 3-6). To be effective, scalers must be sharpened regularly.

Several types of scalers exist (Fig. 3-7). The scaler at the top of Fig. 3-7, commonly called a *sickle scaler,* is most commonly used. The ends of this scaler are mirror images of each other. Depending on the manufacturer, sickle scalers are denoted *H6/7, S6/7,* or *N6/7.* The instrument in the middle is a fine scaler for extremely small teeth. It is known as a *Morris 0-00.* The scaler at the bottom has a sickle scaler on one end and a 33 on the other.

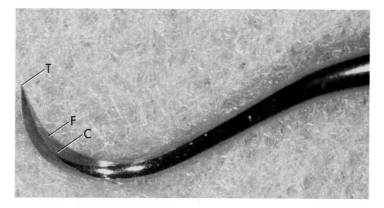

FIGURE 3-6 Parts of a scaler: *F,* face; *C,* cutting edge; *T,* tip.

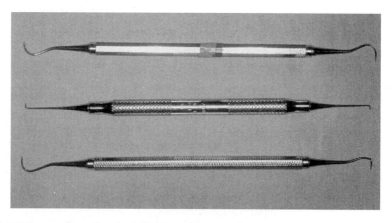

FIGURE 3-7 Three types of scalers: Sickle scaler *(top),* Morris 0-00 *(middle),* and U15/33 *(bottom).*

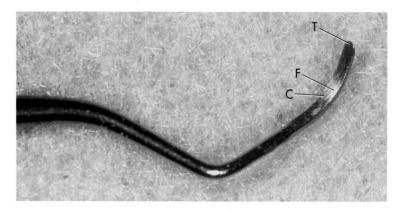

FIGURE 3-8 Parts of a curette: *F,* face; *C,* cutting edge; *T,* toe.

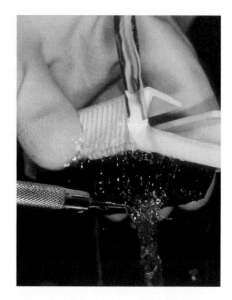

FIGURE 3-9 The instrument should be scrubbed with a brush before sharpening, and heavy duty gloves should be worn.

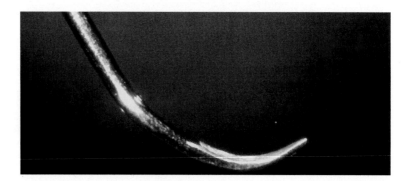

FIGURE 3-10 Because of the dullness of this instrument, the edge can be visualized.

Curettes

Curettes have two sharp sides and a round toe. They are used for the removal of calculus both supragingivally and subgingivally. Curettes are designed so that each end is a mirror image of the opposite end. This allows adaptation to the curved dental surface. If one end does not appear to be adapting to the curvature of the tooth, the instrument can be rotated. There are two types of curettes: the universal curette and the area-specific curette. The universal curette can be adapted to almost all the dental surfaces. The area-specific curette is adaptable to different areas of the mouth. One type of area-specific curette is the Gracey curette. The higher the number of the instrument, the farther back in the mouth it is used.

The point of the curette, called the *toe (T)*, is rounded. The face (F) of the curette is the concave side. The cutting edge (C) is the confluence of the sides and the face. Curettes have a round back (Fig. 3-8).

Curette and Scaler Care

The best practice is to sharpen each instrument after cleaning and disinfecting and before every use. Heavy-duty industrial gloves should be used while cleaning instruments (Fig. 3-9). Alternatively, ultrasonic instrument cleaners may be used. Ideally the operator should have several instrument packs so that the instruments can be cleaned, sharpened, and sterilized between uses. Sterilization reduces the risks of cross-infection among patients and from patients to staff members (e.g., if staff members accidentally injure themselves with the instrument). Disinfecting a stainless steel table before placing an animal on it makes little sense if the instrument itself is unclean.

If an instrument is sharp, its two planes come together at a precise angle. In the past, technicians checked for sharpness by performing the "fingernail" test. For reasons of hygiene, this method is no longer recommended. Visual inspection and sharpening sticks are appropriate methods to check for sharpness.

Testing for sharpness
Visual inspection

All that is needed to perform a visual inspection is a bright light and sharp eye. The instrument is held and rotated toward the light source (Fig. 3-10). If the instrument is dull, the edge is rounded and reflects light. If the instrument is sharp, the edge does not reflect light.

Sharpening stick

A sharpening stick is an acrylic or plastic rod (Fig. 3-11). A syringe casing may also be used to check for sharpness. To test, the edge of the instrument is drawn across the rod. A dull blade glides over the surface without catching at it. Conversely, a sharp blade easily catches as the instrument is drawn against the surface of the sharpening stick.

Sharpening equipment
Flat stone

Several types of flat stones are available for sharpening (Fig. 3-12). The Arkansas stone is used for final sharpening of an instrument that is already close to sharpness. An India stone is used for "coarse" sharpening of an overly dull instrument or for

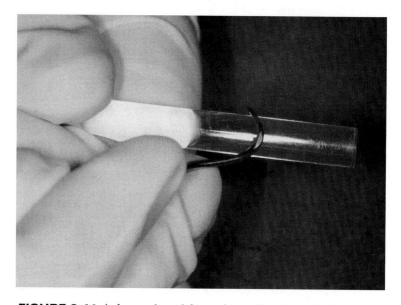

FIGURE 3-11 A sharpening stick may be used to check for sharpness.

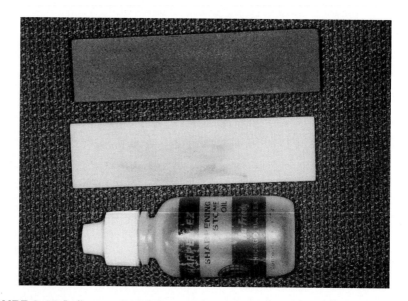

FIGURE 3-12 India stone *(top)*, Arkansas stone *(middle)*, and sharpening stone oil *(bottom)*.

changing the plane of one or more of the sides of the instrument. Sharpening with the India stone is followed by the use of an Arkansas stone. Both the Arkansas and the India stones require oil for effective use. The ceramic stone may also be used for fine sharpening. With ceramic stones, water is generally used as the sharpening medium instead of oil.

Conical stone

A conical stone is a round Arkansas stone. It is used to provide a final sharpening to the instrument by working on its face.

Sharpening technique
Flat stone

Two methods of sharpening with a flat stone are common. One technique is to hold the instrument motionless and move the stone. Because the edge of the instrument is stationary, the blade is highly visible during sharpening. The second method is to move the instrument against a stationary stone (Fig. 3-13). Because the moving stone technique is less difficult, it is the method demonstrated in this text.

A few drops of oil are placed on the sharpening stone (Fig. 3-14). The oil is spread out evenly over the stone with tissue paper. The stone must be lightly coated with oil. The technician must be careful not to wipe off the oil while attempting to spread it. The first step in sharpening the instrument is to hold it firmly against the edge of a table, with the tip facing the operator. The instrument is rotated so that the face *[The face of the instrument is the flat surface between the two cutting edges]* is parallel with the ground. This position provides a reference point for the adaptation of the stone (Fig. 3-15).

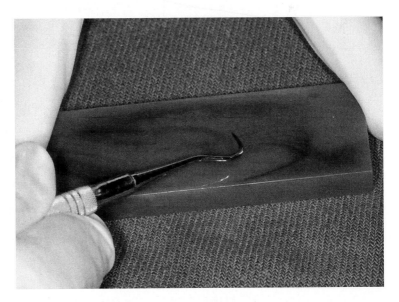

FIGURE 3-13 In this technique the stone is placed on the table or held steady in the hand while the instrument is moved.

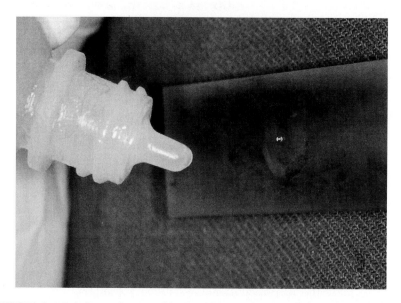

FIGURE 3-14 A drop of stone oil is placed on the stone and spread in a thin layer.

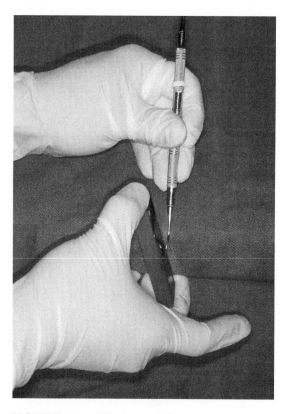

FIGURE 3-15 The instrument is held firmly on the table so that the face is parallel to the ground and the stone adapted to the instrument.

The stone is held with the thumb and index finger at the top and bottom of the stone (Fig. 3-16). The operator should exercise caution: The instrument is sharp and can easily cause injury. The stone is first placed at a 90-degree angle to the face of the instrument, or straight up and down (Fig. 3-17, *A*). The upper portion of the stone is rotated approximately 10 to 15 degrees away from the instrument, or to the 11 or 1 o'clock positions (Fig. 3-17, *B*). This creates a 75- to 80-degree angle at the edge of the instrument.

The stone is moved up and down approximately 1 inch. As the stone is moved down, a "flashing" should be observed on the face of the instrument. The flashing consists of stone oil, stone particles, and instrument particles (Fig. 3-18). As the stone moves up, the flashing should recoat the stone. If the stone is tipped too much (e.g., the top of stone is before 11 o'clock or past 1 o'clock), the stone will miss the convergence of the face of the instrument and the side, and the blade is not sharpened. If the stone is tipped too little (e.g., the top is toward 12 o'clock), the blade may actually become dulled. The sharpening should end on the down stroke, which helps prevent the formation of a bur on the sharpened edge.

Conical stone

The conical stone is rolled over the face (Fig. 3-19). Overuse of this technique shortens the life of the instrument, the strength of which lies in the direction from the face to the back. If the face is removed, the instrument becomes weaker. The advantage of sharpening with a flat stone is that the strength of the instrument is maintained even as the sides of the instrument become worn. The thinning of the flat stone makes it better suited to subgingival work.

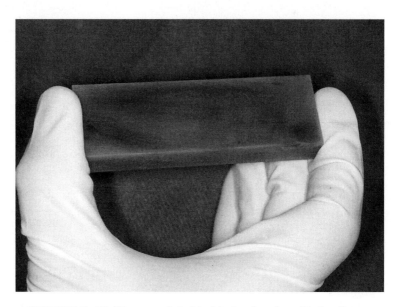

FIGURE 3-16 The stone is held with the thumb and index finger.

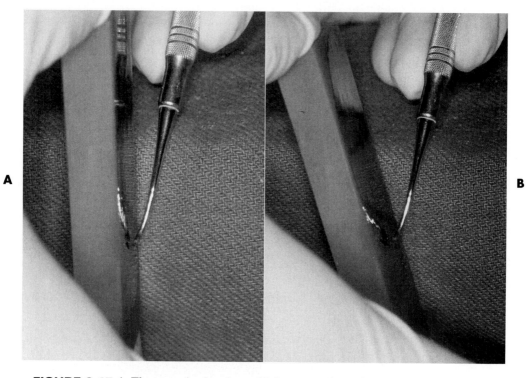

FIGURE 3-17 A, The stone is placed at a 90-degree angle to the face of the instrument. **B,** The stone is rotated approximately 10 to 15 degrees.

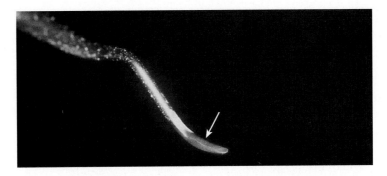

FIGURE 3-18 Flashing on the curette face *(arrow)*.

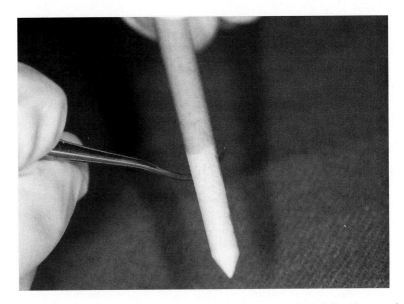

FIGURE 3-19 The conical stone is used by rolling the stone while sliding it toward the tip of the instrument.

POWER SCALERS

Power scalers convert electrical or pneumatic energy into a mechanical vibration (Table 3-1). When the power scaler is placed against calculus, the vibration shatters it, freeing it from the tooth surface. Power scalers operate in the range of 6000 to 45,000 cycles per second. There are three types of power instruments. The ultrasonic scalers work by converting sound waves into a mechanical vibration. The sonic and rotary instruments convert air into mechanical vibration.

TABLE 3-1 Comparison of Mechanical Scalers

Instrument type	Cycles per second	Amplitude (mm)	Active tip (mm)	Motion
Magnetostrictive—metal strips	18,000, 25,000, 30,000	0.01–0.05	5–7	Elliptic
Magnetostrictive—ferroceramic rod	42,000	0.01–0.02	13	Circular
Piezoelectric	25,000–45,000	0.2	3	Linear back and forth)
Sonic	6000	0.5		Elliptic
Rotary			Depends on tip	Circular

Ultrasonic Instruments

Ultrasonic instruments work by converting energy from a power source into a sound wave. This sound wave is picked up at the handpiece. Ultrasonic instruments function in a way similar to that of two identically tuned tuning forks: When one is caused to vibrate, the other starts to vibrate in resonance. Two types of devices in the handpiece can pick up the sound wave and turn it into a vibration. These devices are known as *magnetostrictive* and *piezoelectric* (Fig. 3-20).

Magnetostrictive
Ultrasonic metal strips/stacks
Several manufacturers produce flat metal strip units. These vibrate at 18,000, 25,000, and 30,000 cycles per second. The amplitude of tip movement in these units is between 0.01 and 0.05 mm, which is an extremely narrow motion. Generally, lower amplitudes are better because they cause less damage to the tooth. The working tip is all sides, which results in an uneven motion and an elliptic pattern. Two lengths of inserts are available, which is important to remember when ordering and inserting the inserts into the handpiece (Fig. 3-21).

Ultrasonic and combination electrical motor handpieces
Several of the manufactured dental units are combinations of ultrasonic scalers and electrical motor handpieces. These are used for polishing and simple cutting of teeth. The electrical motor handpieces are generally not as effective as the air-powered high-speed and low-speed handpieces that use compressed air.

Ultrasonic ferroceramic rod
Magnetostrictive ferroceramic rods vibrate at 42,000 cycles per second (Figs. 3-22 and 3-23). These instruments have an amplitude of 0.01 to 0.02 mm with a circular-type motion. All sides of the tip are equally active (about 13 mm of the tip).

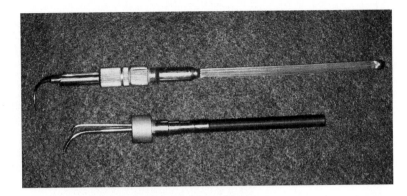

FIGURE 3-20 The magnetostrictive units use either a series of flat metal strips *(top)* or a ferroceramic rod *(bottom)*.

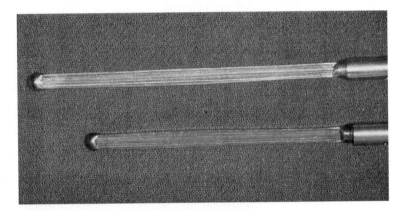

FIGURE 3-21 The longer insert on the top is the 25,000 cycles-per-second (cps) length, and the lower insert is 30,000 cps.

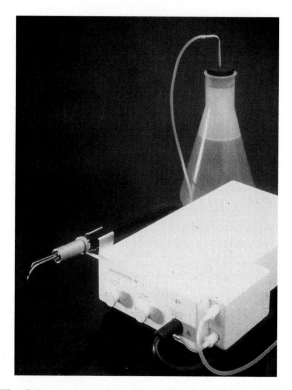

FIGURE 3-22 The Odontoson-M ultrasonic scaler uses a ferroceramic rod. Medicaments such as chlorhexidine gluconate may be placed in the beaker. (Courtesy of Periogene.)

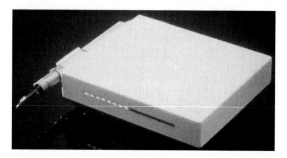

FIGURE 3-23 The Odontoson 5 ultrasonic scaler uses a ferroceramic rod. (Courtesy of Periogene.)

Inserting ultrasonic inserts

If a metal strip/stack unit is used, the unit must be turned on and the handpiece filled before insertion of the insert (Fig. 3-24). However, with ferroceramic rod units the handpiece should be drained before insertion of the insert (Fig. 3-25). Forcing the insert into a handpiece that contains water may cause the tip to fracture.

Piezoelectric

Piezoelectric ultrasonic scalers use crystals in the handpiece to pick up the vibration (Fig. 3-26). The frequency of the piezoelectric units ranges from 25,000 to 45,000 cycles per second. The amplitude of these units is approximately 0.2 mm, which results in a wide, back-and-forth tip motion. Approximately 3 mm of the working tip is active.

Energy nodes

The vibration energy is not distributed evenly down the tip of piezoelectric ultrasonic scalers (Fig. 3-27). The motion of the piezo tip is not uniform. The tip moves farther in one direction than in the other, which means that during use the most active side of the tip must be placed on the part of the tooth where the calculus is to be removed.

Medicaments in irrigating solutions

Many piezoelectric and magnetostrictive units have reservoirs for an irrigating solution. A variety of solutions may be placed in the containers. The most popular and effective solution is 0.12% chlorhexidine. In-line reservoirs may be spliced onto the water line, allowing irrigation solutions to be used in units that do not have their own containers. Another alternative is to use a garden sprayer, otherwise known as a "bug buster," for the water supply. These units must be pressurized by hand.

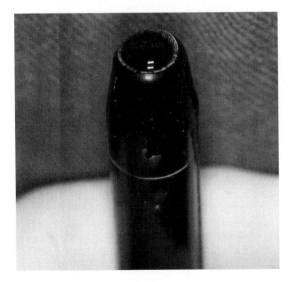

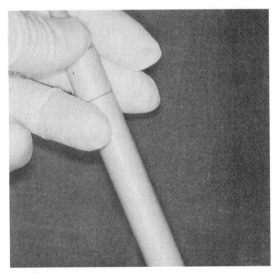

FIGURE 3-24 With a metal strip/stack unit, water should be seen starting to flow out of the tip. This prevents it from overheating.

FIGURE 3-25 With a ferroceramic insert, water is drained out of the handpiece before the tip is inserted.

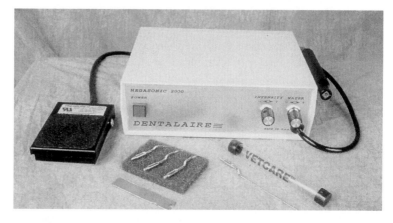

FIGURE 3-26 A piezoelectric ultrasonic scaler. (Courtesy of Dentalaire.)

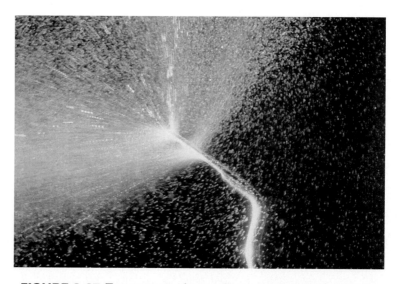

FIGURE 3-27 Two energy nodes are shown on this piezoelectric tip.

Ultrasonic tips

As shown by the tip on the left in Fig. 3-28, the beaver-tail tip is relatively wide. The first type of tip developed, it is used for supragingival cleaning. The middle tip, the "perio probe," is thin and can be used subgingivally. The tip on the right is the furcation tip. Furcation tips hook to the left or right, which allows them to gain access to furcations around crowns and be used subgingivally. Further information on these units and tips is provided in Chapters 7 and 9.

Sonic Scalers

Sonic scalers operate at 6000 cycles per second and have a 0.5-mm amplitude. Their motion is elliptic, in a figure-of-eight motion. All sides of these tips are active during cleaning, although the cleaning action may not be even. One feature of these units is that the compressed air has a cooling effect. They are less likely to cause heat-related damage to teeth than are the ultrasonic scalers.

Air enters the sonic scaler, passes through the shaft, and exits from small holes on the shaft that are covered with a metal ring. The air exits the hole at an angle and causes the ring to start spinning. Because the ring does not fit the shaft tightly, it begins to wobble. This wobbling sets off a vibration that is transmitted down the shaft to the tip (Fig. 3-29).

Rotary Scalers

The use of rotary scalers is discouraged for two reasons. First, rotary scalers can easily damage the tooth. Second, burs must be replaced often because they become dull ex-

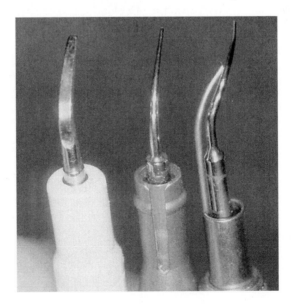

FIGURE 3-28 Ultrasonic tips: beaver-tail tip, perio probe tip, and furcation tip.

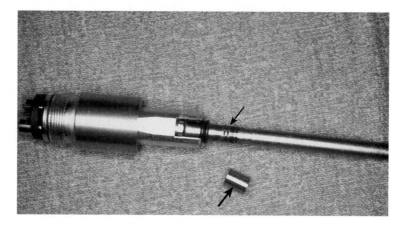

FIGURE 3-29 The cover and vibrating ring of this ultrasonic scaler have been removed. The ring *(large arrow)* covers the two small holes *(small arrow).*

tremely quickly. For proper functioning a new bur must be used for each patient, which is prohibitively expensive.

DENTAL UNITS FOR POLISHING AND DRILLING

Two driving mechanisms exist for polishing and cutting teeth: electrical power and air power. Electrical-powered units generally are the least expensive, although some sophisticated electrical systems, used for specialized procedures such as implantation and endodontics, rival the price of the compressed-air systems.

Electrical-Powered Systems

Electrical-powered systems (Fig. 3-30) operate at lower speeds than air-powered systems and have higher torque. *[Torque. The ability to overcome resistance to movement.]* Except with fairly expensive models, water or irrigating systems cannot be used with electrical-powered systems. Generally, air-powered systems are preferable to electrical-powered systems.

Air-Powered Systems

Two types of air-powered systems exist. One uses compressed gas from a cylinder, the second uses an air compressor. The air compressor pumps air either directly into the dental unit or into a storage tank for slow release to the dental unit. The compressed gas is either room air or nitrogen. Because of associated hazards, oxygen and carbon dioxide should not be used. Oxygen is explosive, and carbon dioxide may be toxic.

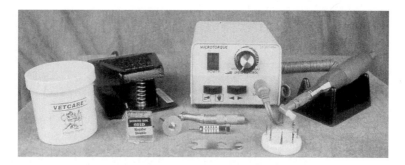

FIGURE 3-30 Electric motor handpiece system. (Courtesy of Dentalaire.)

Air-Compressor Systems

Compressors take the room air and compress it to drive the handpieces. Most units work by pumping air into an air-storage tank. The compressor pumps air into the tank until the pressure inside the tank reaches between 80 and 100 pounds per square inch (psi). At this time the compressor turns off. Air is bled from the tank as it is used by the handpiece at a lower pressure, usually 30 to 40 psi. When the pressure drops below the minimum pressure in the tank, approximately 60 psi, the compressor turns on again, filling the tank back up to 100 psi. Newer compressors are quieter than traditional air compressors. To reduce noise, refrigerator compressors were converted so that they pump air rather than refrigerator coolant. The single-unit compressor rates approximately ½ hp. If a multistation or sonic-scaler handpiece is to be used, a double-unit, 1 hp compressor should be considered. These units are available in portable carts, portable cabinets, and countertop units.

Countertop units allow the unit to be stored in cabinets and other areas remote from the place the procedure is performed. They are self-contained and require only a power source to function (Fig. 3-31).

Dental carts with switches and handpiece holders are available. The compressor may be mounted on the cart or stored in a remote location. The air is connected by hoses (Fig. 3-32). Dental units may also be mounted on walls with the compressor in a remote location, connected by hoses.

Compressor care

Most air-compressor systems use oil for lubrication. The oil level must be monitored frequently because insufficient oil could cause the compressor to cease functioning. Some systems use a dipstick, similar to that of an automobile, for checking the oil. Others have a porthole in the side of the oil reservoir. When adding oil, the technician should always use the type of oil recommended by the compressor manufacturer.

The compression of air into the storage tank may cause condensation. Air-storage tanks have a drain cock that can be turned to let the water out of the tank (Fig. 3-33). Failure to do so allows water to fill the tank, decreasing the effectiveness of the system and possibly ruining the compressor.

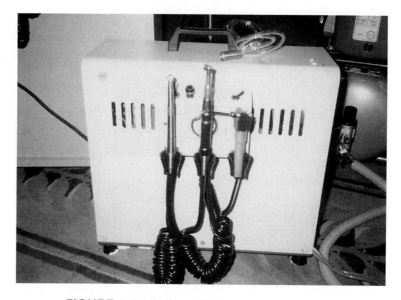

FIGURE 3-31 A silent tabletop compressor system.

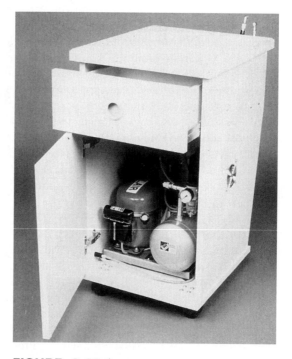

FIGURE 3-32 A cart-type compressor system (Courtesy of Dentalaire.)

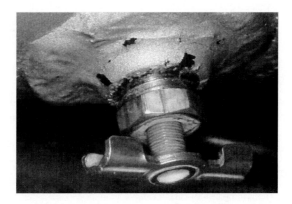

FIGURE 3-33 The drain cock at the bottom of an air-storage tank.

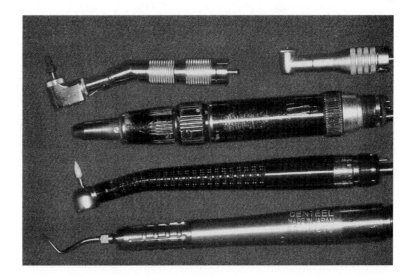

FIGURE 3-34 A variety of handpieces and their attachments: contra angle and prophy angle *(top row);* low-speed handpiece *(upper middle);* high-speed handpiece *(lower middle);* sonic scaler *(bottom row).*

Handpieces

Different types of handpieces can be attached to compressed-air systems (Fig. 3-34). (Sonic scalers have been previously discussed.) Low-speed handpieces are used for polishing with prophy angles and for performing other dental procedures with contra angles. High-speed handpieces are used for cutting teeth in extractions and making access holes into teeth in root canal therapy. All handpieces use a rubber gasket to ensure a water- and air-tight seal. Make sure the gasket is connected when connecting the handpiece (Fig. 3-35).

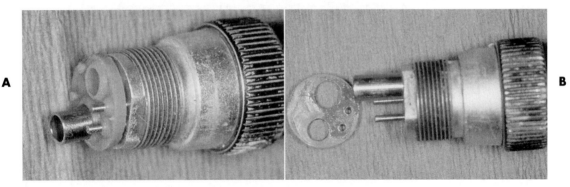

FIGURE 3-35 A, Handpiece with rubber gasket in place. **B,** Handpiece with rubber gasket removed.

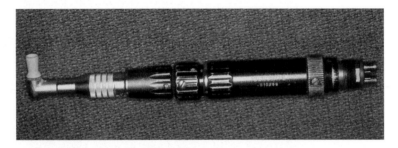

FIGURE 3-36 Low-speed handpiece with prophy angle attached.

Low-speed handpieces

Low-speed handpieces are used for polishing teeth. They have a high torque and a slow speed of 5000 to 20,000 RPM (Fig. 3-36).

Low-speed attachments

A prophy angle is an attachment that allows the use of a prophy cup for polishing teeth during cleaning. (Types of prophy angles and prophy cups are discussed in more detail in Chapter 7.) Attachments are available, such as special files for engine-driven root canals and slow-speed burs for cutting and smooth restoration. A contra angle is an attachment used to change either the direction or speed of rotation (Fig. 3-37).

Care of low-speed handpieces

The low-speed handpiece must be lubricated at the end of each day of use. The technician must first insert lubricant into the smaller of the two large holes, using the oil or spray that comes with the handpiece. WD-40 may be sprayed into the low-speed handpiece once every 2 weeks to remove residues, followed by the recommended lubricant.

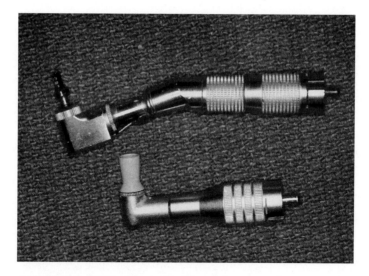

FIGURE 3-37 Prophy angle with prophy cup and contra angle.

Prophy and contra angles

The specific lubrication of prophy and contra angles depends on the instrument. Generally, prophy heads must be lubricated weekly with prophy angle lubricant. For many models the head of the instrument may be twisted off to expose the crown gears that require lubrication (Fig. 3-38). Some prophy angles are self-lubricating. In all cases, the manufacturer's instructions should be consulted for each piece of equipment.

High-speed handpieces

High-speed handpieces turn at 300,000 to 400,000 revolutions per minute. They are used for cutting teeth for exodontics, making root canal entries, and other procedures. Practitioners who use one of these instruments for splitting a tooth in exodontics will find it difficult to return to (or even imagine) the old methods of extracting.

Changing high-speed burs

Two styles of high-speed bur heads are available. One uses a push button on the handpiece to open the chuck. The bur may be removed and replaced by simply pressing the button. The second uses a chuck key. The bur may be loosened and removed by twisting the key counter-clockwise. The new bur is placed in the handpiece, and the bur key turned clockwise to tighten (Fig. 3-39).

Burs should be treated as sharps and disposed of in the sharps container. They should be removed from the handpiece when not in use and when the handpiece is covered. If the bur is removed from the handpiece, a "blank" should be put in its place. If the handpiece is accidentally turned on without a bur in the handpiece chuck, the chuck may be damaged.

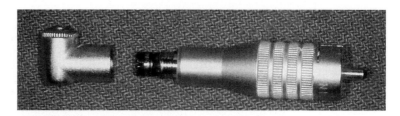

FIGURE 3-38 The head was removed from this prophy angle to show the crown gears.

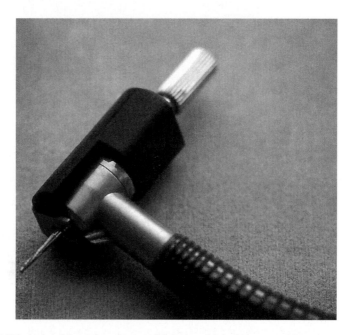

FIGURE 3-39 A chuck key placed over a high-speed handpiece to either remove or replace a bur.

Bur selection

When selecting a bur, the technician must first know the type of handpiece with which the bur is to be used. At the top of Fig. 3-40 is a strait-shank bur that fits directly into the low-speed handpiece. The bur on the lower right is a friction-grip (FG) bur that fits into high-speed handpieces. The bur on the lower left is a right-angle (RA) bur that fits into contra angles for low-speed handpieces. Technicians must be extremely careful when selecting a bur. Some slow-speed FG burs resemble high-speed burs. However, when placed in a high-speed handpiece, these slow-speed FG burs disintegrate under the centrifugal forces placed on them.

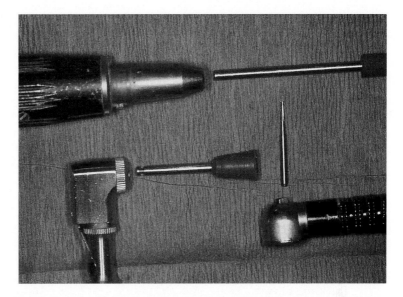

FIGURE 3-40 *(Counter-clockwise)* Straight shaft, friction grip, and right-angle burs.

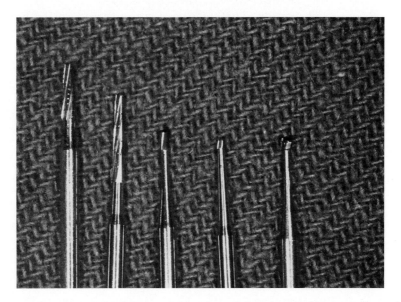

FIGURE 3-41 *(Left to right)* Crosscut fissure, pear-shaped, inverted-cone, and round burs.

Types of burs

Many types of burs have been designed for a variety of uses.

Crosscut fissure burs. The two burs on the left of Fig. 3-41 are crosscut fissure burs, numbered 701 and 701L. The letter *L* indicates a longer cutting surface. The middle bur is pear-shaped, the bur to its immediate right is an inverted cone, and the bur on the far right is round. Crosscut fissure burs are usually numbered in the 500s through 700s. They are used for gaining access to root canals, cutting teeth, and preparing cavities. The crosscut fissure bur is one of the best all-around dental burs. The bur is slightly tapered, with a cutting surface on the side as well as the tip.

Pear-shaped burs. Pear-shaped burs are usually numbered in the 320s through 330s. These burs are a cross between the round bur, crosscut bur, and inverted-cone bur. The result is a bur that has a round cutting tip, cutting sides, and a slight taper for undercutting. It is an ideal all-purpose bur for cavity preparation.

Inverted-cone burs. Inverted-cone burs are usually given numbers in the 30s (e.g., 33 ½, 34, 35). The larger the number, the larger the bur. Inverted-cone burs are used for undercutting in cavity preparation. They are wider at the tip than at the shank.

Round burs. Round burs, numbered ¼, ½, 1, 2, 4, and 6, are general, all-purpose burs. They may be used for access into pulp chambers and for cavity preparations.

Diamond burs. Diamond burs are used for crown preparation (Fig. 3-42). A wide variety of shapes and degrees of coarseness is available. Selection depends on the preparation to be performed.

Finishing burs. A number of burs are used for finishing restorations. One type is a stone, and another has multiple flutes. Fig. 3-43 shows a set of multiple-flute finishing burs.

Care of high-speed handpieces

Lubrication. The high-speed and subsonic scalers should be lubricated daily with a spray-type cleaner and lubricant or another product recommended by the manufacturer of the handpiece (Fig. 3-44, Table 3-2).

Defective turbine. The turbine is the internal portion of the high-speed handpiece that spins at an extremely high speed. It is subject to wear over time and must be replaced periodically. Maintenance may be performed in the office. The signs of a defective turbine cartridge include the following: (1) failure of chuck to tighten around the bur; (2) increased noise or vibration; (3) roughness felt when spinning bur by hand, with turbine in or out of handpiece; (4) intermittent stopping of handpiece; and (5) failure of handpiece to function (Fig. 3-45).

TABLE 3-2
Maintenance Chart*

Procedure	Daily	Weekly	Yearly
Oil in slow speed	√		
Spray in high speed	√		
Check compressor oil level		√	
Drain water out of compressor		√	
Annual compressor maintenance			√

*Manufacturers' recommendations supersede this chart.

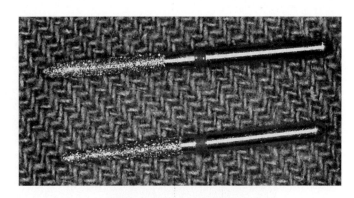

FIGURE 3-42 Diamond burs.

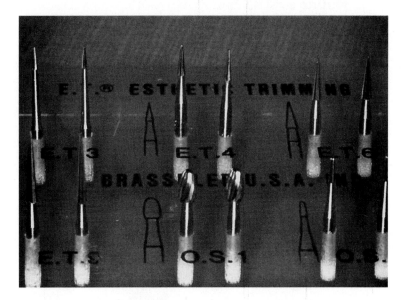

FIGURE 3-43 Finishing bur kit.

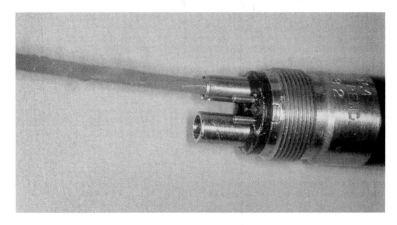

FIGURE 3-44 Lubricating with a spray-type lubricant.

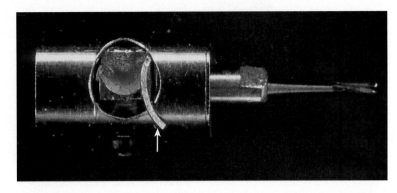

FIGURE 3-45 This turbine was removed from the handpiece. Metal from the inner turbine can be seen protruding from the air exhaust hole.

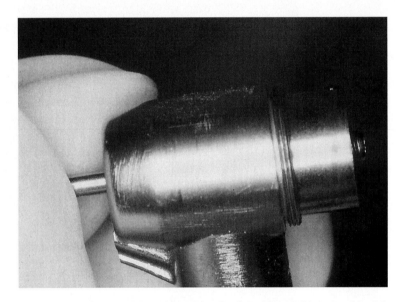

FIGURE 3-46 The turbine is pushed out of the handpiece by pushing on a blank bur in the turbine.

Changing turbines. To change the turbine, a "blank" bur is placed in the handpiece. If the bur that is in the handpiece cannot be removed, caution should be exercised to keep from cutting the hands on the bur. Next, the small metal ring (wrench) supplied with the handpiece is placed on the cap of the handpiece. The handpiece cap is unscrewed and removed by rotating the wrench counterclockwise. The turbine cartridge is removed from the handpiece head by pressing on the blank or bur (Fig. 3-46). The new turbine cartridge is placed into the handpiece head. Finally, the new turbine cartridge is aligned with the pin side up. If the pin is not aligned with the slot, the turbine cartridge will not slide completely into the handpiece head.

Three-Way Syringes

Most dental units come equipped with three-way syringes. These syringes have two buttons. Pressing one button creates a water spray, which can be used to irrigate a tooth surface and clear away prophy paste, tooth shavings, and other debris. Pressing the second button creates an air spray, which can be used to dry the field. The technician must be careful not to flush air into tissues; air can create subcutaneous emphysema or, even worse, enter a blood vessel and create an embolism. Pressing both buttons together creates a mist.

LIGHTING AND MAGNIFICATION

With a few exceptions, the following statement holds true for veterinary dentistry: "If you can't see it, you can't do it." Lighting and magnification are two important aids that allow the technician and practitioner to visualize the structures in the oral cavity.

Lighting is available from a variety of sources. A good surgical light produces wide-ranging, even lighting. Spot lighting is obtained by the use of a light mounted to a headlamp. Focal lighting is achieved by the use of fiber optic lights built into a handpiece.

Binocular eyeglasses produce the best type of magnification. Ideally, they should be adjustable so that the operator's head does not tilt forward; rather, the eyes look down and the head is kept squarely above the shoulders. Three-powered magnification, with a focal length of between 15 and 18 inches, enlarges the subject without excess distortion.

Worksheet

STUDENT NAME: _____

1. The four types of hand instruments are as follows:
   _probe_____ , _explorer_____ , _scaler_____ ,
   _Curette_____ .

2. The portions of all instruments are the handle, the shank, the
   terminal shank, and the _working_____ _end_____ .

3. Color-banded probes have bands that are either
   _____ or _____ mm wide, or a
   combination of the two widths.

4. The newer probe lengths are _____ and
   _____ .

5. Scalers have _three_____ sharp sides and a sharp tip.

6. Scalers are used for _Supragingival_ scaling only.

7. Curettes and scalers are usually _____
   _____ ; this means that they can adapt to opposite
   surfaces.

8. The _____ _____ is the working portion
   of the scaler.

9. The _____ curette may be adapted to almost all the
   dental surfaces.

10. A _____ blade reflects light, whereas a
    _____ blade does not reflect light.

11. The instrument should be sharpened so that it has a
    _____ to _____ degree angle.

12. As the stone is moved down, a " _____" should be observed on the face of the instrument.

13. Powered scalers convert _____ or _____ energy into mechanical vibration.

14. The two following types of devices in the handpiece can pick up the sound wave and turn it into a vibration: _____ and _____.

15. The piezoelectric ultrasonic scalers use _____ in the handpiece to pick up the vibration.

16. Sonic scalers are driven by _____ _____.

17. Handpieces usually operate at _____ to _____ psi.

18. _____ must be periodically drained from air storage tanks.

19. High-speed handpieces operate at _____ speed than low-speed handpieces but have _____ torque than low-speed handpieces.

20. Burs should be treated as _____.

4

Personal Safety and Ergonomics

LAURIE A. HOLMSTROM AND STEVEN E. HOLMSTROM

This chapter discusses occupational safety and ergonomics in the veterinary dental practice.

HAZCOM

The Federal Hazard Communication Standard (HAZCOM, or HCS) is a regulation enforced by the Occupational Safety and Health Administration (OSHA) of the United States Department of Labor. HAZCOM is based on employees' rights and their "need to know" the identities of hazardous substances to which they may be exposed in the work environment. OSHA requires employers to provide workers with preventive safety equipment and ensure that they wear it during dental procedures. To comply with the HAZCOM requirements, employers must also submit a written hazard communication program.

SAFETY REQUIREMENTS FOR VETERINARY DENTISTRY

For the veterinary dentistry practice, OSHA requires that the employer provide safety glasses, masks, and gloves for all employees who perform dental procedures (Fig. 4-1). The employee is responsible for wearing the safety equipment during all procedures. After all, it is the employee's health that is at stake, and flying debris or other substances can easily cause infections if the employee neglects to wear the safety protection provided. Employees must always be careful to take responsibility for their own safety by wearing the necessary safety equipment and should not expect their employers to remind them before each potentially hazardous procedure.

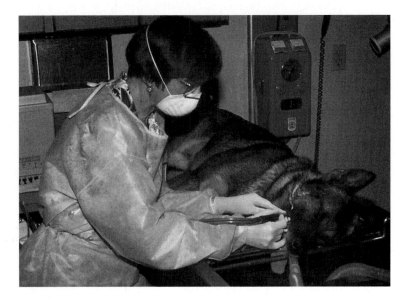

FIGURE 4-1 Minimal safety equipment includes mask, eye protection (preferably a face shield), and gloves.

TYPES OF HAZARDS

Veterinary staff risk exposure to several different hazards. Hazards are classified as follows: chemical, physical, biologic, and ergonomic. Chemical hazards are formulations that can act on the skin, eyes, respiratory tract, alimentary system, and other organs and organ systems. Physical hazards are those that can physically harm. Ergonomic hazards are due to workplace interactions.

EYE PROTECTION

The importance of eye protection cannot be overstated. Infections from a number of sources can cause permanent visual impairment. Unprotected operators are sometimes struck in the eye by pumice while polishing or by a flying piece of tooth during high-speed drilling. Scaling can also send bacteria-laden calculus into the dental technician's eyes or mouth. The calculus almost always scratches the eye and thereby deposits bacteria directly into the wound. Splatter from rinsing acid etch or sodium hypochlorite is potentially devastating to the eyes and can also cause small lesions on the face.

MOUTH AND LUNG PROTECTION

Use of high-speed equipment, such as ultrasonic scalers and high-speed drills, creates a vapor that contains bacteria, blood, saliva, and tooth dust. This vapor extends up to 3 feet from the source and can irritate and infect the respiratory system of people who are not wearing protective masks. The risk extends to nonemployees, such as clients visiting the dental area while a procedure is in progress.

Masks

Respirator masks offer more protection than surgical masks. All masks must fit tightly to function properly. Some allow for adjustments at the upper (nose) and lower (chin) portions of the mask.

HAND AND SKIN PROTECTION

Gloves protect the patient from cross contamination and protect the veterinary staff from the toxic materials used in dentistry. Toxins in resins, such as methyl methacrylate, formaldehyde, chloroform, x-ray chemicals, and cold sterilization chemicals, are all absorbed through the skin. Some are carcinogenic and accumulate in the body with repeated exposure. Most affect the liver and kidneys. Because of the critical importance of these organs, all staff members should wear proper safety protection when handling these materials.

HAND WASHING

Proper hand washing is important for disease control. If employees do not wear gloves and are accidentally stabbed by an instrument or bitten by a patient, they may become infected by the organisms on their own skin. Employees should always wash their hands before putting on gloves in case a glove is torn or otherwise penetrated during the course of a procedure.

Hand-Washing Agents

A number of hand-washing agents are available. Simple anionic detergents (soaps) help by destroying the cell walls of bacteria. Antiseptics such as alcohol, iodine, iodophors, and hexachlorophene are also effective. The ability of chlorhexidine, parachlorometaxylenol, and triclosan to stick to surfaces, a property known as *substantivity,* makes these agents superior.

Hand-Washing Technique

Proper technique in hand washing is important. Rings and other jewelry (e.g., bracelets) should be removed. Hands should be washed for a minimum of 1 minute immediately on arrival to the office and then washed again for 15 seconds between each patient.

Employees should rinse their hands in cold water, making sure to remove all soap. Then, they should dry their hands thoroughly. Many people rinse their hands in hot water, mistakenly believing that if it hurts, it is killing bacteria. In fact, the hot water causes the pores in the hands to open, which draws water from the hands and makes them more susceptible to dermatitis.

GLOVE CONCERNS

Some people develop allergies to latex gloves with time. Three types of hypersensitivity reactions to latex exist. The first is known as a *contact urticaria*. It is an immediate, Type I allergic reaction that occurs immediately after exposure. Contact urticaria manifests itself as hives, nasal inflammation, general itching, and wheezing. The second type is a systemic reaction, also known as a Type I reaction, and results in conjunctivitis, asthma, and systemic anaphylaxis. The fact that latex powder remains in the air for a long time if gloves are snapped on complicates the reaction. The third type is a contact dermatitis, which is a delayed, Type IV allergy. It causes a localized rash and develops 24 to 72 hours after exposure. Because many conditions mimic these hypersensitivities, employees should consult an allergist if they experience problems.

Proper fit in gloves is also important for preventing hand fatigue that can lead to tendonitis in the wrist. Gloves should be loose through the palm of the hand. If they are too tight, the muscles of the palm will cramp with the effort to maintain a relaxed position.

SHARPS

Needles are another source of potential infection. To keep from accidentally stabbing themselves, employees should never recap needles with both hands. The needle should be scooped up with one hand (Fig. 4-2) or simply discarded in the sharps container. Sharps containers should be disposed of properly when they reach the full line. To prevent punctures when inserting needles, employees should never continue to pack additional needles in the containers after they are full.

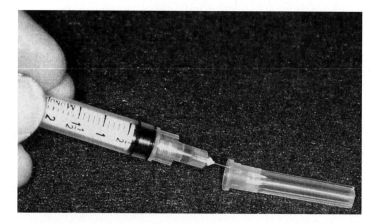

FIGURE 4-2 The scoop technique should be used to recap needles.

EYE SHIELDS

Light-curing guns use an intense white light to cure resins. Because looking at the light can cause permanent retinal damage, employees should use the approved orange shields and refrain from looking at the light except when necessary.

SAFETY WITH PRODUCTS

Employees should always know the materials in the products used for all procedures. Reading the instructions and following them carefully are crucial steps for safety.

Material Safety Data Sheets

Chemical manufacturers and importers must convey hazard-related information to employers by means of labels on containers and material safety data sheets (MSDSs). In addition, all employers are required to implement a hazard communication program to provide this information to employees. Methods for educating employers include container labeling, MSDSs, and training sessions. Employers must receive sufficient information to design and implement employee protection programs. HAZCOM also provides necessary hazard information to employees so that they can participate in and support the protective measures instituted in their workplaces.

Labels

All hazardous materials in original containers must bear a label from the manufacturer that is legible, in English, and prominently displayed on the container. The following information must be included:
1. Product identity: trade name, product name, or chemical identity
2. Appropriate hazard warnings: physical and any relevant acute or chronic health hazards
3. Name and address of the chemical manufacturer, importer, or other responsible party

Composite Restoration Materials

Most composite restoration materials require an acid etch for maximal adhesion. This solution, which can splatter when rinsed off, is extremely strong and can cause damage if it touches an area other than the enamel. In addition, chemical reactions to the uncured resins are possible. Acid etch should be used with caution. Employees should always wear gloves and glasses and understand the proper way to use this substance.

Amalgam Restoration Materials

Amalgam restoration materials contain mercury, which can be absorbed into the skin and, if left in open containers, vaporize. Excess amalgam should be stored covered with water or x-ray fixer in a closed container. Employees should never touch amalgam with bare skin.

Toxins

Toxic chemicals, radiographic chemicals, disinfectant surface cleaners, ultrasonic cleaning solutions, and cold-sterilizing chemicals should never be handled without gloves. The toxic substances that cause them to work are absorbed through the skin and can accumulate in the body, causing major health problems in the future. The solutions used in ultrasonic instrument cleaners are not necessarily sterile, and bacteria can enter the hand through small cuts and openings.

REPETITIVE MOTION DISORDERS

Repetitive motion disorders are prevalent in occupations that require repeated small repetitions of a single action. Dental hygienists and computer operators are particularly susceptible to this problem. Veterinary technicians who work exclusively in dentistry are therefore at risk.

Symptoms include stiffness in the neck and shoulders (particularly on the dominant side), soreness in the elbow and/or wrist, hand fatigue, headaches, and tingling or numbness in the fingers of the affected side. Tendonitis may also occur in the elbow and wrist as a result of bad positioning. These symptoms often decrease or disappear completely with increased attention to positioning, stroke and hand placement, ergonomics, and strengthening exercises. Occasionally the damage to the nerves is so extensive that the technician is no longer able to work in dentistry at all.

Ergonomics in the Workplace

Prevention of repetitive motion disorders is based on keeping repetitive motions as stress-free as possible. Ergonomics is the science of designing the workplace so that operators remain in the most neutral positions possible.

Neutral position

A neutral position entails sitting with the knees slightly below the hips, the back straight, the elbow at a 90 degree angle, and the thumb relaxed at the top of the hand. The head points straight forward, and the shoulders are relaxed. Feet should be flat on the floor or resting on a full footrest on the chair. The back is as straight as possible, with the head leaning over as little as possible (Fig. 4-3). While working, the employee should be careful to keep the shoulders relaxed (not hunched) and the head level, neither tilted too far forward nor leaning toward either side. (The head weighs 12 pounds and is supported only by the small column of the neck.) Dental personnel should never lean on the table supported by their forearms or bend the wrist from the straight position. A bar rest for the feet provides inade-

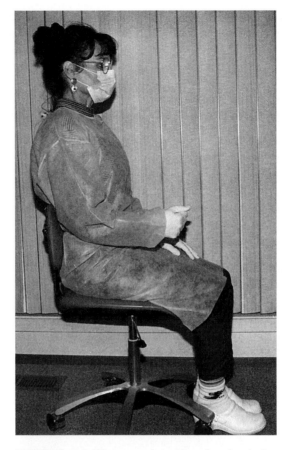

FIGURE 4-3 The neutral position: head pointing straight forward, shoulders relaxed, back straight as possible, and feet on the floor.

quate support for the lower back; resting the feet on the floor with too great an angle between the hips and knees also puts pressure on the lower back and impairs circulation to the lower leg and feet. The working motion while hand scaling should be a pull stroke that rolls the entire forearm, bending the wrist as little as possible.

Preventive procedures

Repetitive stress injuries can be prevented in a variety of ways. The types of instruments used can make a significant difference. Use of ultrasonic scalers and hand instruments with the correct types of handles helps. Patient positioning is also relevant. Selecting the correct glove size and regularly performing hand-strengthening exercises are also important preventive measures.

Fitted gloves versus ambidextrous gloves

The use of ambidextrous gloves can cause fatigue. The thumb may be pulled back to a nonneutral position, which exerts excessive force on the thumb as it moves forward (Fig. 4-4). Left and right gloves keep the thumb in a neutral position (Fig. 4-5).

Mechanical dentistry

Use of mechanical-powered dental instruments in place of manual hand instruments reduces the risk of injury. Mechanical-powered dental instruments should therefore be used whenever possible. Ultrasonic scalers are an excellent choice for removal of heavy deposits and subgingival root cleaning; these instruments eliminate the need for all but the most cursory scaling.

Instrument handles

Because instruments with "fat" handles are easier to hold, they reduce the fatigue caused by pressing the handles with sufficient force to remove deposits (Fig. 4-6).

Patient positioning

Sandbags are used to position the patient for easy access and visibility, which also improves the operator's positioning. Use of a dental operating light rather than a surgical light affords greater flexibility in illuminating the deeper parts of the mouth so that the operator does not need to lean excessively to see the back teeth. Technicians should remember that during the course of a procedure they can change their own position or the position of the patient to reduce the risk of injury. Some teeth

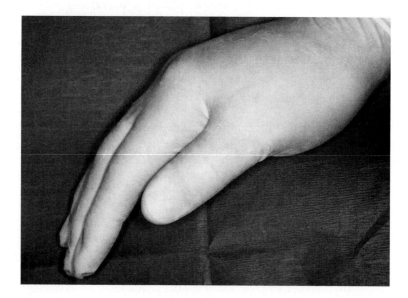

FIGURE 4-4 Some manufacturers claim that their gloves work equally well on both hands, but this is not true. These ambidextrous gloves pull the thumb back, creating stress.

are more easily reached from over the head, some from the front of the mouth, and some from the patient's mandible side.

Strengthening exercises

Strengthening the muscles opposite the ones used in dental procedures reduces stress on the working muscles by providing more overall support. Employees should remember to stretch during long procedures or whenever they feel fatigued. Alternating hand and mechanical procedures during treatment also helps rest muscle

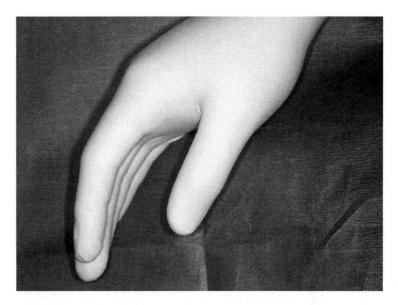

FIGURE 4-5 This glove is specifically designed for the right hand. Note the less fatiguing neutral position.

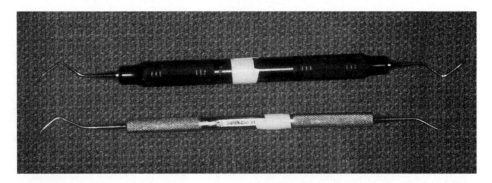

FIGURE 4-6 The instrument on the top has a "fat" handle, which is preferable; the bottom instrument has a thin handle.

groups. To relax the shoulders in a standing position, employees can interlace their fingers behind their backs and raise them up as high as possible while leaning forward slightly. This position should be held for 30 seconds (Fig. 4-7).

Another simple way to relax the shoulders while working is to sit up straight, with the hands parallel against the sides. Then, the thumbs should be turned outward as far back as possible while the stomach muscles are tightened. This position should be held for 30 seconds (Fig. 4-8).

To relax the back, the employee should interlace the fingers overhead, with the palms toward the ceiling. With the feet approximately hip width apart and the arms at ear level, the employee should then lean first to the right for 30 seconds and then to the left for another 30 seconds (Fig. 4-9).

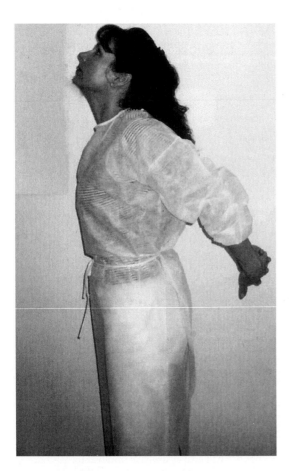

FIGURE 4-7 Back shoulder stretch.

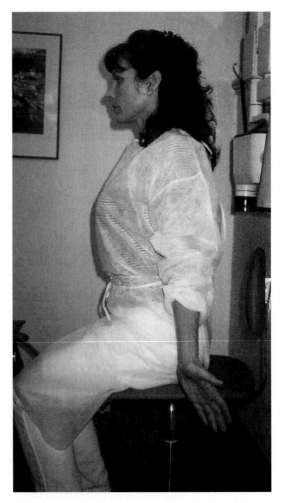

FIGURE 4-8 Side shoulder stretch.

To stretch the forearm muscles, employees should raise one arm almost straight forward and then pull their index, middle, and ring fingers back until they feel resistance, taking care not to lock the elbow. This position should be held for 30 seconds (Fig. 4-10).

To stretch the opposite muscles, employees should bend the hand downward, gently push against the fingers, and hold for 30 seconds (Fig. 4-11). Performing these last two exercises several times a day is recommended, particularly when the technician is especially fatigued (e.g., after scaling the teeth of a patient with an unusual amount of calculus).

Lifestyle Ergonomics

Attention to muscle groups used in dentistry must also extend into life outside the workplace. Employees should give their bodies a chance to heal and rest between workdays. Regular exercise that does not repeat the same motions frequently per-

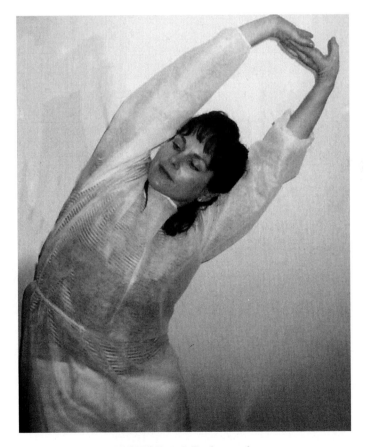

FIGURE 4-9 Back stretch.

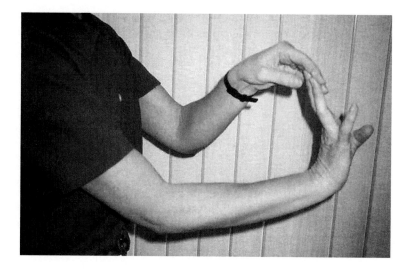

FIGURE 4-10 Forearm stretch.

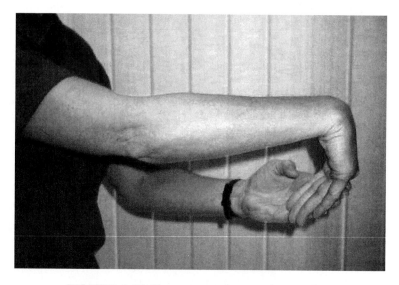

FIGURE 4-11 Forearm stretch, opposite muscles.

formed at work is a good way to maintain health and general well-being. Employees should make an effort to work opposing muscle groups and acquire balanced muscle development as well as working out regularly to relieve the stresses of the day.

Power walking is one of the better ways to maintain overall body toning and relieve stress without overusing injury-prone areas. Using light hand weights (1 pound) while power walking also helps develop upper-body strength without stressing the neck or wrist areas. Heavy Hands® handles without weights on them allow carrying weight without the need to hold onto them (no "squeeze factor"). Wrist weights also work as long as they are not tight or moving up and down on the wrist. They should always be carried with the arms bent at a 90-degree angle; straight arms exert pressure on the elbow tendons.

Preventing injury away from the workplace

Performing small-motor activities, such as needlework, prevents the muscles and tendons from relaxing sufficiently after work. Over time, muscles may become sore or irritated. Certain forms of exercise, such as bike riding, put pressure on the wrist, lower back, and neck in much the same way that dental procedures do. Consequently, the body does not have the opportunity to recover from the stresses of the workplace. Carrying heavy items, such as shopping bags, luggage, and large purses, stresses the elbow and wrist tendons excessively and can also cause neck and shoulder pain. Using suitcases with wheels, making frequent trips to deposit shopping bags in the car, and carrying a small purse with only the necessities all help relieve these problems.

Sleeping with the hands curled into the pillow irritates the wrist tendons. People who habitually do this should try tucking their hands flat under the pillow before falling asleep or purchasing braces that hold the wrists in a straight position. These braces should be worn at night until the habit of bending the wrists is broken. Sleeping on the side or back (rather than on the stomach) is also much better for the neck and shoulders. Although sleeping habits are hard to break, the reduction in neck pain makes the attempt worthwhile. Neck-support pillows (the kind that have a depression in the middle) keep the neck in a good position during sleep. The average working life of a dental hygienist who sees 8 to 10 patients a day 4 days a week is 5 to 6 years; after that, repetitive motion disorders force the hygienist to decrease his or her workload. Any measures to reduce stress and promote proper alignment in injury-prone areas lengthen the employee's professional life and reduce the pain caused by repetitive motions.

Worksheet

STUDENT NAME: _____

1. Employers are required by _____ to provide employees with preventive safety equipment and require them to wear it during dental procedures.

2. Employees must always be careful to take responsibility for

   _____ _____ _____.

3. Hazards are classified as follows: _____,

   _____, _____, _____.

4. Scaling can also send _____-laden calculus into the dental technician's eyes or mouth.

5. Proper _____ is important for disease control.

6. Employees should be careful to rinse their hands in

   _____ water.

7. A Type I allergic reaction takes place _____ after exposure.

8. Chemical manufacturers and importers must convey hazard information to employers by means of labels on containers and

   _____ _____ _____

   _____.

9. The ultrasonic solutions are not _____ and contain bacteria that can enter the hands through small cuts and openings.

10. Attention to muscle groups used in dentistry must also extend into life _____ the workplace.

5
Anesthesia

MEGHAN RICHEY AND CHARLES MCGRATH

Two weeks ago Mrs. Humphry brought Mitzi to the veterinary dentistry practice for her annual visit. Mitzi, a 14-year-old toy poodle, is the center of Mrs. Humphry's life since her husband passed away several years ago. The entire staff likes Mrs. Humphry and Mitzi; Mitzi is a sweet dog, and Mrs. Humphry follows the staff's every recommendation regarding Mitzi. Mrs. Humphry was initially reluctant to schedule an appointment to have Mitzi's teeth cleaned because she feared the effects of the anesthesia on a dog of Mitzi's advanced age. However, both the technician and the veterinarian reassured Mrs. Humphry that performing blood work and an electrocardiogram (ECG) before the procedure would ensure Mitzi's safety. Last week Mitzi's blood panel and ECG were found to be within normal limits for a 14-year-old poodle, and the procedure was scheduled for today.

This morning anesthesia was induced and maintained according to the usual protocol for the practice. Approximately 5 minutes after turning Mitzi to clean her other side, the technician noticed that Mitzi was no longer breathing and her tongue was blue. The veterinarian, who was performing surgery, removed her gloves quickly and performed CPR. Despite these efforts, Mitzi could not be revived and was pronounced dead. The veterinarian had to return to the incomplete surgical procedure, and the technician knew that Mrs. Humphry was sitting by the telephone, waiting for a call regarding Mitzi.

Informing clients that their pets died during elective dental procedures recommended by the veterinarian not only is difficult but also endangers the reputation of the practice. The following sections discuss anesthesia as it applies to dental patients.

ASPECTS OF ANESTHESIA

All aspects of anesthesia are important. With regard to dental procedures, the following are especially crucial:
1. Airway management
2. Patient monitoring and support

3. Attention to airway management
4. Pain management
5. More attention to airway management

The veterinarian determines most aspects of anesthetic case management (e.g., selection of the patient, preoperative test choices, drug selection), but the technician also plays a vital role in the safety and outcome of the procedure.

The following sections review various aspects of respiratory anatomy and physiology that are vital to the provision of high-quality anesthetic care.

RESPIRATORY PHYSIOLOGY REVIEW

Most technicians are not respiratory physiologists, but they should have a basic understanding of proper airway management. Because the lungs and associated structures are essential for gas anesthesia, knowledge of the basic concepts and terminology is necessary.

The main purpose of the respiratory tract (or lungs) is to deliver oxygen (O_2) to the blood and eliminate carbon dioxide (CO_2) that was produced by the peripheral tissues. Gas exchange occurs in the alveoli, and the process of breathing (specifically termed *alveolar ventilation*) replenishes gases for exchange with blood by diffusion across the alveolar-capillary membrane. However, O_2 and CO_2 are **not** equally diffusible; nor are they interchangeable in the evaluation of respiratory function.

Several factors control and regulate breathing (or ventilation) in the awake animal. Voluntary control, often for the purpose of vocalization, can affect an animal's breathing, but breathing is usually rhythmic and involuntary as a result of interactions and feedback from various neural centers (known as *respiratory centers*) in the brain. These respiratory centers establish the rhythm of breathing. Because respiratory centers are subject to the effects of anesthetics, the breathing rhythm changes during anesthesia. Although the respiratory centers still control the rhythm, O_2 and CO_2 become much more important influences in determining the actual rate and depth of breathing.

Oxygen is an important respiratory stimulant, with the role of "coarse" adjustment. If oxygen levels in blood fall, the impulse to breathe increases. By comparison, CO_2 can be considered respiratory "fine tuning," with the ability to make subtle adjustments to the breathing rate. Respiratory responses to even subtle changes in CO_2 levels in blood are extremely rapid because the chemoreceptors are much more sensitive to changes in CO_2 than to changes in O_2. In most animals under anesthesia, CO_2 tends to be the primary stimulus for breathing: Increasing levels of CO_2 stimulate breathing so that it is faster and deeper; decreasing levels of CO_2 suppress breathing so that it is slower and more shallow. The term *ventilation* therefore refers to CO_2 removal, not to O_2 delivery. CO_2 measurement is the benchmark for assessing alveolar ventilation partly because arterial CO_2 is principally influenced by its rate of production (metabolic activity) and its rate of elimination (alveolar ventilation).

$$\frac{\text{Production (aerobic metabolic activity)}}{\text{Elimination (alveolar ventilation)}} = PaCO_2$$

Good ventilation (i.e., normal CO_2) is possible with poor O_2 transport (i.e., low O_2). Conversely, O_2 levels may be adequate even in the face of moderate hypoventilation or increased CO_2.

Gas exchange occurs as follows: CO_2 leaves the blood and enters the alveoli of the lung much more rapidly (i.e., about 20 times faster) than O_2 crosses the alveolar wall into the blood. After crossing the alveolar-capillary membrane, O_2 binds to hemoglobin in the red blood cells. The time a red blood cell spends in a pulmonary capillary adjacent to alveoli is about ¾ of a second. The combination of the short time frame and the differences in solubility between the two gases means that O_2 blood levels are much more likely than those of CO_2 to be adversely affected by respiration changes or a pathologic condition (Box 5-1). The terms *hypoxia, hypercapnia,* and *hypocapnia* mean low blood O_2 levels, high blood CO_2 levels, and low blood CO_2 levels, respectively. Gases (e.g., CO_2, O_2, isoflurane, halothane) travel according to concentration gradients (more accurately termed *partial pressure gradients*), moving from an area of high concentration or partial pressure to an area of lower concentration or partial pressure. All things being equal, the larger the gradient (i.e., the higher the "high" or the lower the "low"), the faster the gas will move.

Gases are measured a bit differently than other substances and, to add to the confusion, may be measured in several different ways. Although the actual amount of O_2 (or CO_2) in milliliters of O_2 per 100 milliliters of blood is important, measuring this amount is not feasible. Instead, either the partial pressure of each gas or the percentage of saturation of hemoglobin by a gas (usually only O_2) is measured. Partial pressure is measured in millimeters of mercury (mm Hg), also known as *torr.* Partial pressure is the portion of atmospheric pressure that is exerted by the gas being measured. At sea level, atmospheric pressure is 760 mm Hg. Humidity in the air accounts for approximately 45 to 50 mm Hg of the pressure; the resultant 710 mm Hg is the sum of all the partial pressures of the gases in room air. Room air is 21% oxygen; 21% of 710 mm Hg is 140 mm Hg. The partial pressure of O_2 in room air is therefore 140 mm Hg. In awake patients breathing room air, the partial pressure of O_2 in the alveoli or arterial blood is actually only about 100 mm Hg because of the partial pressure of CO_2 in the alveoli (about 40 mm Hg; $140 - 40 = 100$). In the perfect animal with perfect lung function, alveolar and arterial partial pressures are equal.

BOX 5-1
Causes of Hypoxia and Hypercapnia

Causes of hypoxia	Causes of hypercapnia
Hypoventilation	Hypoventilation
Low inspired O_2 concentration	Ventilation/perfusion mismatch
Ventilation/perfusion mismatch	
Shunts (right to left)	
Diffusion impairment (alveolar)	

Determining the percent hemoglobin saturation of oxygen is another common means of quantitating O_2 levels of blood. Percent hemoglobin saturation is different from partial pressure, although the terms are often confused and interpreted as the same piece of information. Hemoglobin saturation measures the percentage of hemoglobin that is bound with O_2 (100% being the maximum percentage). Unlike most relationships, the relationship between hemoglobin saturation and oxygen partial pressure is not linear but sigmoid (Fig. 5-1). As such, a one-to-one relationship between hemoglobin saturation and O_2 content or O_2 partial pressure does not exist. A saturation of 100% corresponds to an O_2 partial pressure of 100 mm Hg (or more); 90% saturation corresponds not to 90 mm Hg but rather to 60 mm Hg; and at a hemoglobin saturation of 50%, the O_2 partial pressure is only 25 mm Hg.

The terminology used in respiratory physiology is often confusing at first. The following phrases are used when describing the gases' locations in the lung and the pulmonary tree. The breathing apparatus of an animal includes not only the lungs but also the conducting airways. These conducting airways include the mouth, nose and sinuses, pharynx, larynx, trachea, main stem bronchi, and each successive branching of the bronchi down to the bronchioles (Fig. 5-2). These structures contain inhaled (or exhaled) gases, but these gases do not take part in O_2/CO_2 exchange. Gas exchange occurs **only** in the alveoli.

When a normal breath is taken, the amount inhaled is called a *tidal volume.* In the normal animal, this is 10 to 15 ml/kg (5 to 7 ml/pound) of body weight. However, as previously stated, not all of this tidal volume participates in gas exchange. Normally, only two thirds of each breath enters the alveoli for participation in gas exchange, and the remaining one third fills the conducting airways. The two thirds of the tidal volume is the alveolar ventilation because it removes CO_2 from the alveoli. The remaining third within the conducting airways is called *anatomic dead space,* or *dead*

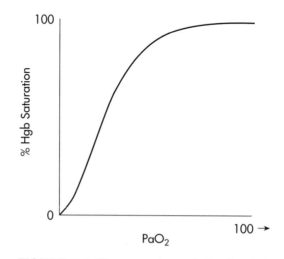

FIGURE 5-1 The oxygen-hemoglobin dissociation curve. The scales on the *X* and *Y* axes are the same. Note that when the PaO_2 is greater than 100 mm Hg, the percentage hemoglobin saturation remains at 100%.

space for short. A second form of dead space (gas that is inhaled or exhaled but does not take part in gas exchange), called *physiologic dead space,* is composed of alveoli that are not eliminating CO_2. In normal patients the two types of dead space should be the same if normal alveoli are present. Changes in dead space affect ventilation (i.e., CO_2 levels) but can also affect O_2 and inhalant levels. The importance of dead space will become clear when endotracheal tubes and other equipment are discussed.

Two other frequently used terms often used are *vital capacity* and *functional residual capacity (FRC)*. Vital capacity is the **most** a patient can inhale (or exhale) (i.e., a deep breath or a heavy sigh). It is usually about 5 times a regular tidal volume. FRC is the amount of gas left in the lungs after a normal exhalation. Its purpose, other than to prevent lung collapse between breaths, is to provide for gas exchange between breaths. Because the heart continues to pump blood between breaths, blood still passes through the pulmonary vasculature to eliminate CO_2 and pick up O_2.

One final area of respiratory physiology that is important in anesthesia is resistance to breathing. During a normal breath, gas is drawn in rapidly through the trachea, which is a wide tube. With each branching of the pulmonary tree, the size of the airway decreases and the resistance to the airflow increases. This slows the speed of gas entering the alveoli to a mere trickle. If, however, the tracheal lumen is narrowed (i.e., blocked by a foreign body or a mass), the initial resistance to gas flow increases, making breathing more difficult for the patient. Resistance increases relative to several factors, as defined by Poiseuille's law:

$$\text{Resistance} = \frac{8\,n\,L}{\pi\,r^4}$$

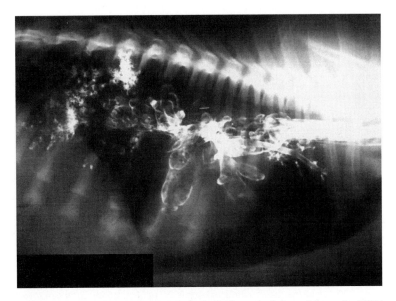

FIGURE 5-2 Bronchogram of a dog. Organic iodine was injected into the ETT and aspirated, outlining the conducting airways distal to the tip of the ETT: distal trachea, mainstem bronchi, and sequential branching of bronchi to bronchioles and terminal bronchioles.

where L is the length of the trachea and r is the radius. Therefore any reduction in the radius of the airway is **inversely** related to the resistance because $R \sim 1/r^4$. Because the radius is to the fourth power, a 50% reduction in the radius results not in a doubling of the resistance but rather in a sixteenfold increase. A 25% reduction equals a threefold increase, a 33% reduction equals a fivefold increase, and so on. However, doubling the length through which the patient is breathing also doubles the resistance because $R \sim L$. In normal patients the airway lumen is large enough to reduce resistance but not so large that it increases dead space volume.*

For a more complete yet concise review of respiratory physiology and pathophysiology, *Respiratory Physiology* and *Respiratory Pathophysiology*, by John B. West, MD, PhD, are both excellent.

Commonly Used Abbreviations

P_aO_2, S_pO_2, and F_IO_2 are all commonly used abbreviations in physiology. The first letter, always in upper case, represents **what** is being measured (i.e., **P**artial pressure, **S**aturation, **F**raction, respectively). The second letter, subscript upper or lower case, represents **where** the measurement is being made. Lower-case letters indicate liquids, and upper-case letters are gas related (i.e., **a**rterial, **v**enous, **p**eripheral, **c**apillary and **A**lveolar, **E**xpired, **T**idal, **I**nspired, **B**arometric). The third set of letters and numbers represents the gas being measured (i.e., O_2 for **O**xygen, CO_2 for **C**arbon dioxide, N_2 for **N**itrogen).
Therefore:

P_aO_2 = partial pressure of arterial oxygen
P_AO_2 = partial pressure of alveolar oxygen
F_IO_2 = fraction of inspired oxygen
S_pO_2 = saturation of peripheral oxygen
$P_{ET}CO_2$ = partial pressure of end (or expired) tidal carbon dioxide (also often written as $_{ET}CO_2$)
V_T = volume tidal (i.e., tidal volume)
V_D = volume dead space (or dead space volume)

AIRWAY MANAGEMENT

Protection and maintenance of a patent, secured airway is essential to a successful outcome for the dental patient. Because anesthetized patients are unable to protect

---

*The following three methods demonstrate the effect of reducing the radius by 50%, 25%, and 33%: 50% is 0.5. $1/0.5^4 = 16$. Or $1/0.5 = 2$ and $2 \times 2 \times 2 \times 2 = 16$. Or, the inverse of 1/2 is 2/1 (or 2), $2^4/1^4 = 16/1 = 16$.
25% reduction is 75% of original size. 75% is 0.75. $1/0.75^4 = 3$. Or $1/0.75 = 1.33$ and $1.33 \times 1.33 \times 1.33 \times 1.33 = 3$. Or, the inverse of 3/4 is 4/3, $4^4/3^4 = 265/81 = 3$.
33% reduction is 67% of original size. 67% is 0.67. $1/0.67^4 = 5$. Or $1/0.67 = 1.49$ and $1.49 \times 1.49 \times 1.49 \times 1.49 = 5$. Or, the inverse of 2/3 is 3/2, $3^4/2^4 = 81/16 = 5$.

their airways, aspiration is a major concern. Even basic hand scaling poses the risk of tartar, debris, and water entering the patient's airway. When an ultrasonic scaler is used, large volumes of water flood the pharyngeal area, and the patient may aspirate water or loosened debris. In awake patients the spray results in swallowing, gagging, or coughing.

Because of these risks, all animals undergoing dental procedures should be intubated with a cuffed endotracheal tube (CETT) (Fig. 5-3). Contrary to popular belief, dissociative-based anesthetic protocols (e.g., ketamine HCl, Telazol®) do not maintain protective airway reflexes. Patients under dissociative-based anesthesia still swallow, cough, gag, and move their tongues but not necessarily as protective reflexes; use of injectable anesthetics does **not** ensure a patent, protected airway.

Airway Protection

Adherence to the following guidelines ensures an adequately protected airway from induction through recovery.

1. **Use cuffed endotracheal tubes only** (Fig. 5-4).
2. **Check each cuff before induction** of the patient. Gently but fully inflate each cuff, remove the syringe, and allow the cuff to remain inflated for 10 to 15 minutes to ensure the absence of a slow leak in the cuff, pilot tube, or pilot balloon. The cuff should inflate evenly and symmetrically. Before fully deflating the cuff, gently squeeze and hold the cuff for a moment. This mimics the conditions that

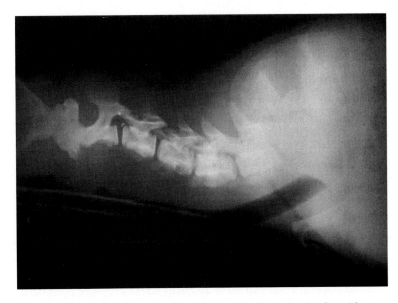

FIGURE 5-3 Radiograph of a properly positioned endotracheal tube with a properly inflated cuff.

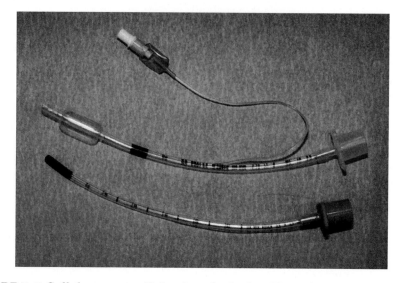

FIGURE 5-4 Cuffed versus uncuffed endotracheal tubes. The endotracheal tube on top is cuffed, with its high-volume/low-pressure cuff fully inflated. The endotracheal tube on the bottom is uncuffed.

the inflated cuff will have in the trachea and ensures that no leak is present when pressure is applied to the cuff. Then **fully** deflate the cuff. If the cuff fails any of these steps, it should be removed from service and replaced or repaired.

3. **Select three different CETT sizes**—one that you think will fit the patient, one a size smaller, and one a size larger. Endotracheal tubes are sized in millimeters (in half-millimeter increments) by their internal diameter, or ID. The outside diameter, or OD, is dependent on wall thickness and varies according to the type of tube. Therefore the same patient may require tubes of different sizes depending on the type selected (Fig. 5-5). Use the largest size that will **comfortably** fit the patient's trachea. Fully deflated cuffs and use of a water-soluble lubricant (e.g., K-Y® jelly) facilitate comfortable passage of maximum-diameter tubes. Using the largest comfortable tube size is important because larger tubes fill the trachea more completely, reducing the risk that fluids and debris will enter the lungs should the cuff fail.

4. **Secure the endotracheal tube.** This step is frequently overlooked. When securing the tube, most technicians are careful to tie the gauze securely around the patient's nose or head; however, they are not always careful to ensure that the gauze around the tube is snugly secured. When the gauze is loosely knotted, the tube can slide back and forth within the loop. Although a loose knot makes removal of the gauze from the tube much easier at cleanup, a loose knot does not secure the tube to the patient.

5. **A cuff sealed to 10 to 20 cm of water pressure** is sufficient to prevent water from passing the cuff in a recumbent dog, with its head either level or lower than its body (Fig. 5-6). Such a seal allows positive pressure ventilation for periodic "sighing" or "bagging" of the patient and also prevents excessive pressure from being

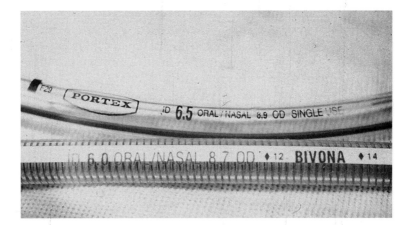

FIGURE 5-5 Both these tubes fit the same dog. The top tube has an ID of 6.5 mm and an OD of 8.9 mm. The bottom tube has an ID of 6.0 mm and an OD of 8.7 mm. If the top tube was used during a previous anesthetic and then the bottom tube was used during a subsequent anesthetic, a 6.5-mm (ID) tube from the manufacturer of the bottom tube would not fit the patient because of a larger OD.

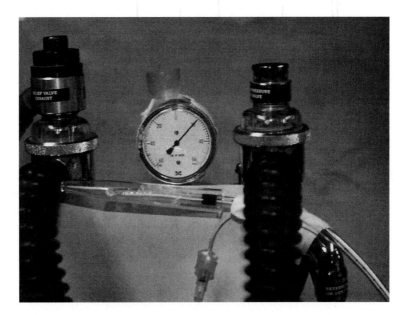

FIGURE 5-6 A CETT tube inflated within a clear test tube, with the circuit adjusted to 20 cm of water pressure (on the circuit manometer). The pop-off valve *(far left)* is closed, and the pressure is maintained at 20 cm of water.

applied to the tracheal mucosa, which reduces the risk of the formation of tracheal mucosal edema after extubation. The formation of edema after extubation reduces the size of the tracheal lumen and, according to Poiseuille's law, results in increased resistance to airflow. Clinically, this phenomenon manifests itself as stridor after extubation.

6. Another frequently neglected step is **packing the oropharynx.** Packing the oropharynx with 4×4 gauze prevents debris from entering the pharynx, larynx, and trachea cranial to the cuff. The gauze also serves as a second line of defense should the seal of the cuff become loose during the procedure. When packing the oropharynx, be sure to use a large piece of gauze, preferably 4×4 or laparotomy sponges. Small pieces of gauze (e.g., 3×3 or 2×2) or cotton balls are sometimes left behind after extubation, resulting in airway obstruction during recovery. Attaching a string to the packing materials serves as a visual reminder to remove the packing at the end of the procedure. If a string is not used, be sure to record at the time of packing the number and size(s) of packing materials used. This information can be noted in the record or, better yet, on a piece of tape applied to the patient's head.

Techniques of Intubation

The following steps are guidelines for proper intubation.

1. **Select tubes of appropriate sizes and with functional cuffs.**
2. **Ensure that the tube is the proper length.** Many practitioners use tubes as they come out of the package, which means that there is only one length of tube for each tube size. This results in excessively long tubes, especially in smaller patients. Endotracheal tubes may also be too short, but only in the unusual event that the cuffed section does not extend beyond the larynx.
3. **Intubate promptly once adequate anesthetic depth has been achieved.** Visualize the larynx and arytenoids, and gently insert the tube between them. Timing the passage of the tube with inhalation reduces trauma to the arytenoids, especially in cats.
4. **Connect the patient to the anesthesia machine promptly, and quickly check the patient's vital signs:** presence of pulse and its character and rate (the lingual approach is usually most convenient), eye reflexes and position, mucous membrane color and refill time, and so on. Any detected abnormalities can be corrected now before they become a crisis. If the machine has not been previously primed and filled with oxygen and inhalant, inflate the reservoir bag and give the patient a breath of oxygen. A minute or more may elapse before the patient breathes on its own, depending on the induction technique used. During this time the heart is pumping blood through the lungs. Without this first breath or two of oxygen, the oxygen concentration in the alveoli drops rapidly from 21% (room air), which causes hypoxemia, a life-threatening condition. The initial breath of 100% oxygen fills the lungs with a higher concentration of oxygen, making hypoxemia less likely. The initial apnea is often due to the rapidly delivered high concentration of induction drug(s), which suppresses the respiratory center. However, if the patient is only lightly anesthetized at the time of intuba-

tion, apnea may still occur. In fact, some lightly anesthetized patients voluntarily hold their breath.

5. **Secure the tube to the patient firmly** to prevent tube movement and slippage (see item #6 under Airway Management).

6. **Inflate the cuff.** Most mistakes are made during inflation. The usual technique is to draw some volume of air into an empty syringe, pump this air into the cuff via the pilot balloon, and then try to judge the adequacy of the seal by the feel of the balloon (Fig. 5-7). Then, once the technician is satisfied with the feel of the pilot balloon, the cuff is forgotten until it is time to deflate the cuff at extubation. This approach is **incorrect.** A properly inflated cuff provides an airtight seal only to an airway pressure of 10 to 20 cm water. The following steps will accomplish this.

Note: The technician's hand should never be removed from the pop-off exhaust valve from the time it is closed until it is reopened.

a) Be sure the cuff is not yet inflated. Close the pop-off valve, and gently squeeze the bag to a pressure of 10 to 20 cm of water. Put your ear near the patient's mouth, and listen for air leaking around the cuff while watching the manometer rise toward 20 cm of water. Another approach is to watch the manometer to see if the pressure holds steady at 10 to 20 cm of water while squeezing the reservoir bag. If the anesthesia machine does not have a manometer or a non-rebreathing system is being used (Fig. 5-8), the technician must develop a feel for the pressure in the bag using the hand. Now, open the pop-off valve.

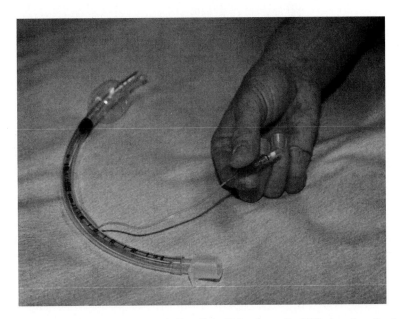

FIGURE 5-7 Fully inflated (i.e., overinflated) cuff that has a "soft" feel to the pilot balloon; if this were in a patient, the addition of more air would be incorrectly thought necessary based on the pilot balloon.

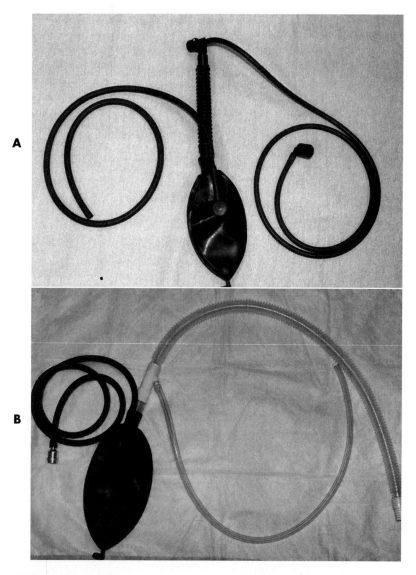

FIGURE 5-8 Two commonly used nonrebreathing systems. **A,** Norman elbow: Fresh gas enters via tube on the right; the "pop-off" valve is the black disc on the reservoir bag that covers the exhaust hole in the bag; the hose on the left goes to scavenge system for evacuation of waste gases. **B,** Bain's coaxial system: Fresh gas enters via the clear tube; exhaust gas leaves via the reservoir bag and black hose (as with the Norman elbow).

b) If there was no leak, the seal is adequate by virtue of the correct tube size. However, a leak is more likely.

c) To properly inflate the cuff, attach an air-filled syringe to the pilot balloon valve. Repeat steps *a* and *b* while gradually adding air to the cuff until no leak occurs at a pressure of 10 to 20 cm of water.

d) Open the pop-off valve.

The assumption that a good seal has been achieved for the duration of the procedure is natural but incorrect. As the level of anesthesia deepens and the patient's muscles relax, the trachealis muscle also relaxes (Fig. 5-9). After 15 to 30 minutes, the internal diameter of the trachea is larger than it was at intubation. The seal should be checked again at this time and additional air added if necessary.

Airway Complications

No procedure or technique is without some risk or potential problem, and intubation is no exception. Adhering to the previously discussed guidelines can generally prevent intubation-related problems. The following section addresses the reasons that these guidelines are necessary.

1. **Why use the largest-diameter tube possible?**
   a) The larger the tube, the less air is needed to inflate the cuff to form a seal. Cuffs are one of two types: high-volume/low-pressure and low-volume/high-

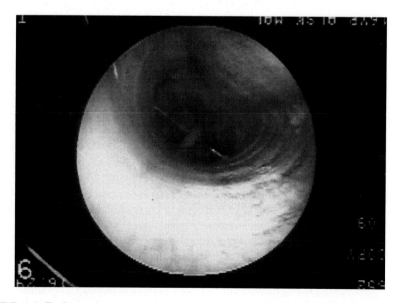

FIGURE 5-9 Endoscopic view of a trachea. The carina is visible, at a distance, in the center. Cartilage rings can be seen from 2 o'clock to 12 o'clock *(clockwise)*. The slightly bulging tissue between 12 o'clock and 2 o'clock is the relaxed trachealis muscle.

pressure. Portex® and other plastic disposable tubes have high-volume/low-pressure cuffs. These cuffs hold a large volume of air with minimal pressure in the cuff, producing a softer cuff to seal against the tracheal mucosa. As the cuff inflates, it spreads so that it is in contact with a larger surface length of the trachea without exerting much pressure against the tracheal mucosa. However, as the cuff reaches its maximum volume, the pressure in the cuff increases dramatically and transfers to the tracheal mucosa. This pressure on the tracheal mucosa significantly increases the risk of ischemic damage and associated complications after extubation.

Overinflation of high-volume/low-pressure cuffs also sometimes results in rupture of the cuff or occlusion of the Murphy eye (Fig. 5-10) of the endotracheal tube, increasing the risk of airway obstruction should the tip of the tube become occluded. The Murphy eye, which is the hole in the side of the tube between the cuff and tip, is designed to provide an alternate avenue for gases should the tip become lodged against the wall of the airway or otherwise occluded.

Bivona® and Magill® (red rubber) tubes are low-volume/high pressure cuffs (Fig. 5-11). These cuffs hold a smaller volume of air but at a much higher pressure. They are designed to inflate to their full lengths with only a small volume of air. Because the cuff expands very little, a properly fitting tube is essential to form a competent seal with the tracheal mucosa. As more air is added, the pressure within the cuff (which is therefore applied to the tracheal mucosa) increases tremendously. When this cuff type is overinflated, ischemic damage is likely to occur. Moreover, the combination of a high-pressure cuff; a soft, pliable endotracheal tube wall; and rigid tracheal rings can also result in collapse of the endotracheal tube, resulting in airway obstruction.

b) Resistance to airflow is another important reason to use as large a tube as feasible. Smaller-diameter tubes are more difficult for the patient to breathe through because of the increased resistance, as Poiseuille's law demonstrates. In the case of endotracheal tubes, the radius (r) is the inside diameter of the tube (diameter = radius $\times$ 2). Because of the thickness of the walls of the endotracheal tube, the radius of the patient's trachea decreases during intubation. Therefore tubes with a large internal diameter (or internal radius) should be used to minimize the reduction in radius and the increase in airflow resistance.

2. **Why should the technician verify that the tube is not too long and does not extend beyond the patient's incisors?** Long tubes cause three problems, which are described as follows:

a) The resistance to airflow is increased (as previously discussed).

b) Dead space increases. Dead-space gas is high in CO_2 and low in O_2. In anesthetized patients, dead space should be increased only by the volume of the wye piece. (The corrugated hoses, tubing, reservoir bag, CO_2 absorbent canister, and other parts of the anesthetic circuit do not contribute to dead space if the unidirectional valves are functional.) When the CETT extends beyond the incisors, dead space increases. In small patients, this increase is often significant, causing more of the inspired gas to be dead-space gas (i.e., previously exhaled gas) rather than fresh gas. Hypercapnia, hypoxia, and a lightened

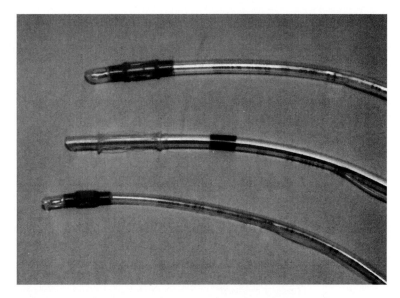

FIGURE 5-10 Three CETTs. The top and bottom tubes each have a Murphy eye; the middle tube does not.

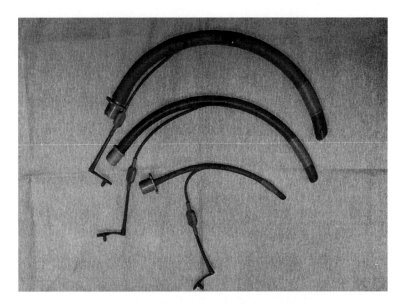

FIGURE 5-11 Examples of Magill tubes. Notice the absence of a check valve, where a syringe is attached to inflate the cuffs. As such, the pilot tube must be occluded by pinching off an area between the syringe and the pilot balloon. The port is then capped before release of the occlusion.

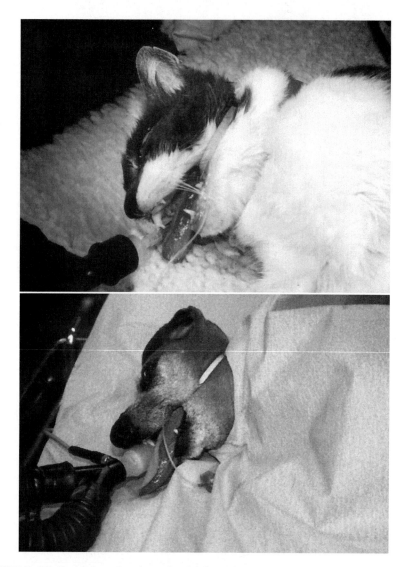

FIGURE 5-12 Examples of endotracheal tubes of proper length. The endotracheal tube connectors are at or near the patients' incisors. Notice that both endotracheal tubes are secured with rubber bands, reducing the likelihood of the tube moving during the procedure.

plane of anesthesia may result. A properly fitting endotracheal tube should not extend beyond the patient's incisors (Fig. 5-12).

c) When long tubes are used, the excessive tube length must either protrude from the animal or be inserted beyond the carina. If the latter occurs, endobronchial intubation and one-lung anesthesia result (Fig. 5-13). Hypoxemia and possible death may follow. The trachea bifurcates at the level of the base of the heart, at

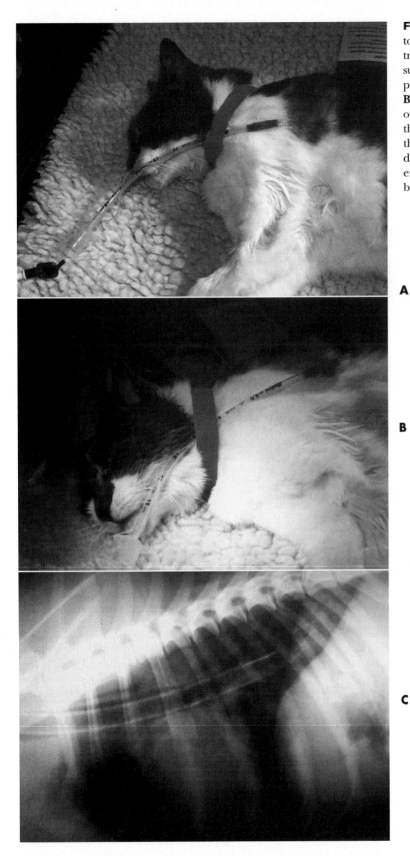

FIGURE 5-13 A, CETT that is too long, with the excess protruding from the patient; this results in an increase in this small patient's dead space volume. **B,** CETT that is too long: no part of the tube is protruding, but the excess would be at or past the carina. **C,** Radiograph of a dog with an excessively long endotracheal tube in a mainstem bronchus.

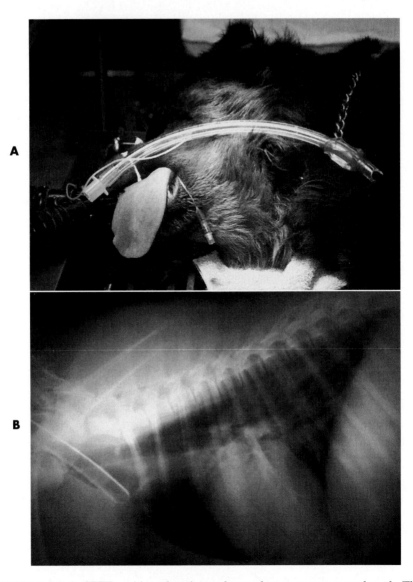

FIGURE 5-14 A, CETT positioned against a dog to demonstrate proper length. The connector is at the dog's incisors, and the tip is just at the thoracic inlet or shoulder joint. (Note that the "real" endotracheal tube has slipped into the dog's mouth past his incisors. If this tube were a bit long for the patient, endobronchial intubation could result.) **B,** The tube shown is the correct length, but it is in the esophagus; it obviously did not go between the arytenoids.

approximately the fifth or sixth rib. When the tube is measured, the tip should reach the thoracic inlet or only slightly beyond (Fig. 5-14).

2. **What happens if the endotracheal tube slips slightly during the procedure and the technician pushes it back in or the technician repositions the patient and does not disconnect the CETT from the anesthesia circuit?** Tube movement within the trachea damages the tracheal mucosa, often to the point of laceration or rupture. Movement of even a partially inflated cuff can result in significant damage to the tracheal wall by the shearing and tearing forces applied by the cuff to the tracheal lining. This effect is most common in cats and small dogs because they have friable, delicate tracheal mucosa and trachealis muscles. If the tube does not move very much, the animal may merely cough for a few days. If the endotracheal tube requires repositioning, the cuff should be deflated before the tube is moved. Patients should **never** be moved, turned, or otherwise repositioned while attached to the anesthetic circuit. The rotation of the patient around the cuff, or rotation of the cuff within the patient, acts as a rotary bur, stripping the mucosa from the tracheal rings. Patients must always be disconnected from the circuit before they are moved, repositioned, or turned.

PATIENT MONITORING

The monitoring of patients during dental procedures is often inadequate. Unfortunately, most dental patients are older animals who would benefit from careful monitoring. Although technicians are usually working near patients' heads, where monitoring is easy, they tend to become preoccupied with the task at hand. Compounding the problem, the wet environment and patient movement (by the technician) cause unreliable readings in many electronic monitors. As a result, the most critical patients are often monitored the least. Monitoring may be broken down into three categories (with some overlap): anesthetic depth, cardiovascular, and respirator.

Anesthetic Depth and Maintenance

The ideal anesthetic depth for dental procedures is often difficult to achieve. Procedures performed vary from nonstimulatory (e.g., routine scaling of normal teeth) to extremely painful (e.g., extraction of teeth, root canal therapy). As a result, the level of anesthesia can suddenly change from too light to too deep.

Eye position (Fig. 5-15), the presence or absence of palpebral and oral reflexes (swallowing, gagging, tongue movement), jaw tone, and quality and rate of the lingual pulse are useful indicators of anesthetic depth and easily observed during dental procedures. An understanding of the concepts of minimum alveolar concentration (MAC), potency, and solubility as they apply to the inhalant anesthetic being used helps in the determination of an appropriate vaporizer setting (Table 5-1). However, vaporizer settings should always be tailored to the individual patient, never just set and forgotten.

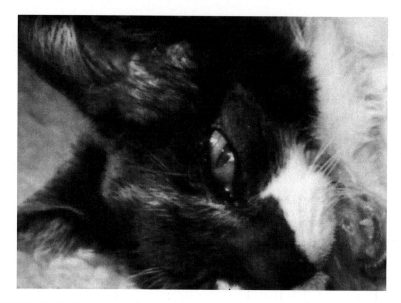

FIGURE 5-15 Stage 3, plane 2 anesthesia, as indicated by the ventrally rotated eye.

TABLE 5-1 **Properties of Inhalant Anesthetics**

	Methoxy-flurane	Halothane	Isoflurane	Enflurane	Sevo-flurane	Desflurane
MAC	0.3%	0.9%	1.3%	2.1%	2.3%	7.2%
Potency	Most	→	→	→	→	Least
Solubility (blood-gas)	15	2.54	1.46	2.0	0.68	0.42
Vapor pressure	23	244	239	172	160	669

Cardiovascular Monitoring

The most commonly used methods of cardiovascular monitoring, from simplest to most complex, are as follows:

Palpation of peripheral pulses
Auscultation of heart sounds
Esophageal stethoscopes
ECG monitor
Pulse oximetry (Fig. 5-16)
Noninvasive blood-pressure (NIBP) monitoring
    Doppler ("Parks") (Fig. 5-17)
    Oscillometric ("Dinamap")
Direct blood-pressure monitoring

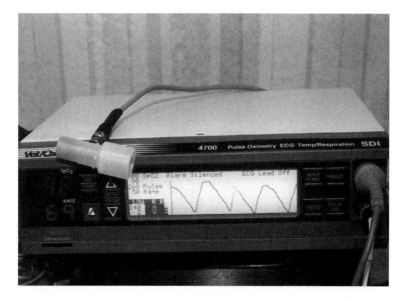

FIGURE 5-16 Multifunction monitor. At the time this photo was taken, the pulse oximetry probe was attached to a patient. A wave form is generated with each pulse, as well as digital readouts of the SpO$_2$ (98%) and pulse rate (69) at the far left.

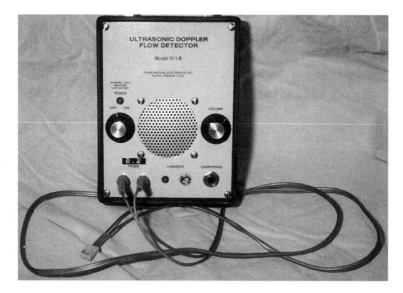

FIGURE 5-17 Parks Doppler: speaker and piezoelectrode. A blood pressure cuff with a manometer and insufflation bulb are necessary to achieve a blood-pressure reading.

Each method has advantages and disadvantages, a detailed discussion of which is beyond the scope of this chapter. However, technicians should be familiar with the monitors used in their practice and should know their capabilities, limitations, and causes of false readings. Certain problems with cardiovascular monitoring are unique to dental procedures. Patient movement is common and can wreak havoc on ECG electrodes, pulse oximetry probes, and NIBP cuffs, producing artifacts and setting off alarms. Patient movement can also cause arterial lines to become dislodged. Because technicians are working in patients' mouths, lingual pulse oximetry probes can be awkward and esophageal stethoscopes pick up external noise from the ultrasonic scaler and high-speed drills, making heart and breath sounds difficult to hear. However, because most dental patients are older animals, attention to cardiovascular monitoring is imperative so that the veterinarian can intervene early, before a crisis develops. Covering the patient protects ECG electrodes, and pulse oximetry probes may be placed on many sites besides the mouth (e.g., flank, web of the hock, between the toes, under the tail).

Respiratory Monitoring

Like cardiovascular monitoring, respiratory monitoring entails use of both simple and sophisticated techniques and instruments:

Observation of the thorax and reservoir bag for coincidental movement (Fig. 5-18)
Auscultation of the thorax for breath sounds
Esophageal stethoscope

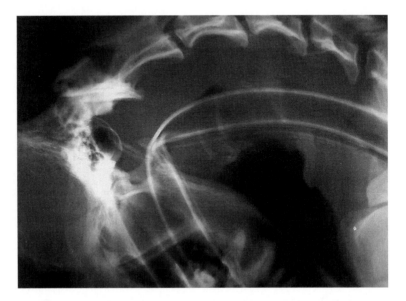

FIGURE 5-18 Radiograph of a dog. Its flexed neck has resulted in kinking of the endotracheal tube and a complete airway obstruction. Without intervention, this dog's chest would continue to rise and fall, albeit with significant effort. However, the reservoir bag would not move with the dog's attempts to inhale and exhale.

"Apnea" monitors (flow detectors)
Pulse oximetry
Plethysmography

Regardless of the method used, observation of coincidental movement of the patient's thorax wall and the reservoir bag is essential. As with cardiovascular monitoring, each method has advantages and disadvantages, which cannot be discussed in detail in this text. In general, however, external noise interferes with auscultation methods, pulse oximetry probes become dislodged when applied to the tongue, and patient movement creates interference that makes plethysmograph readings unreliable.

A more common problem regarding respiratory function, however, is not related to monitoring but rather to compression of the chest wall caused by the technician leaning against the patient or using the thoracic wall as an equipment stand. Even in large dogs, the pressure applied by an arm or elbow can significantly restrict inspiratory efforts; in smaller patients, it can prevent inspiration altogether. Because older patients have reduced muscle strength, not much weight is required to exceed their intercostal muscle capacity.

PATIENT SUPPORT

All too often, patient support is neglected, in part because many dental procedures take relatively little time. However, several factors make patient support during dental procedures as important, if not more important, as it is in more invasive procedures.

Patient Positioning

Most dental patients are placed in a head-down, laterally recumbent position. Although this position allows water to drain from the patient, it also allows abdominal viscera to fall forward onto the diaphragm, impeding its caudal movement, which is necessary for effective inspiration. Care should be taken not to elevate the patient's hindquarters any higher than necessary. Often, merely packing the oropharynx eliminates the need to tilt the patient. Occasional "sighing" or "bagging" of the patient may be necessary, especially if the patient is positioned head down, to reinflate the lungs. Atelectasis of the lower lung occurs even in laterally recumbent patients (Fig. 5-19). When the patient is then turned to the other lateral recumbent position (left to right or right to left), the original atelectatic (lower) lung is placed up and the new dependent lung starts to become atelectatic. During this time the lungs may not be able to exchange oxygen, and a hypoxic crisis may develop soon after changing the patient's position.

Patient Thermoregulatory Control

Dental patients are as susceptible as surgical patients to hypothermia. Dental patients are usually placed on either racks/grates or unprotected, hard, cold surfaces

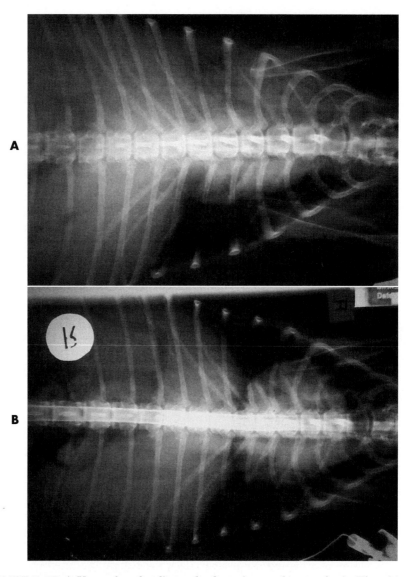

FIGURE 5-19 A, Ventrodorsal radiograph of a patient under anesthesia. The white area to the patient's right is collapsed or atelectatic lung, and without the inflated lung holding it in normal position, the heart has shifted to that side. **B,** The same patient after several manual breaths to reinflate the lungs. Note that both sides of the thorax are the same and the heart is once again centrally positioned, with both the left and right lungs fully inflated. (Courtesy of Dr. Colin Carrig.)

to facilitate drainage of the water used during the procedure. Even if towels are placed over or under the patient, they rapidly become wet, which further contributes to patient cooling. External heat sources are seldom used because of the hazards (e.g., electric shock, thermal burns) they pose in this wet environment (Fig. 5-20). Because dental patients are often older animals, their thermoregulatory capacity is less than that of the normal young adult. Older patients may have less body fat, lower metabolic rates (possibly hypothyroidism), less muscle mass to generate heat by shivering, and thinner skin, all of which contribute to more rapid body cooling.

In addition, vasodilating drugs are commonly used during most anesthetic periods, including dental procedures. Premedication with acetylpromazine (or "ace"), even in low to minuscule doses, produces profound vasodilatation (and hypotension). Halothane, isoflurane, and other inhalant anesthetics are among the most potent vasodilators known. Vasodilatation enhances loss of body heat and contributes significantly to hypothermia.

As a result, particular attention must be paid to keeping the patient as warm and dry as possible and preventing further heat loss. Use of an impervious drape to cover the patient helps keep the patient dry. Use of synthetic fleece or other materials that wick moisture away from the surface helps maintain a dry surface beneath the patient and also helps keep the patient dry.

Use of low-flow anesthesia and a circle system helps conserve heat and humidity in the inspired gases, further reducing heat loss. With nonrebreathing systems, use of a coaxial system (e.g., Bain's system) helps warm the inspired gas. Remember, however, that low-flow anesthesia is **not** an option with a nonre-

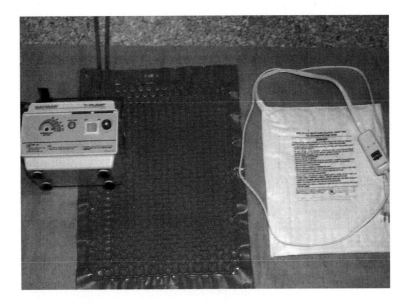

FIGURE 5-20 Circulating warm water blanket and pump *(left)* and electric heating pad *(right)*. The water blanket is safer and will not cause thermal injury to recumbent patients.

breathing system. Warmed IV fluids also help maintain body temperature near normal. However, caution must be exercised to ensure that the fluids are not too hot, especially if a microwave oven was used. The bag must be agitated to mix the hot inner fluid with the cooler outer fluid before the administration set is attached. In small patients the flow rate is low enough that even previously warmed fluids will cool to room temperature before reaching the patient. Coiling the IV line near the patient in a pan of hot water or under a heating pad aids in rewarming the fluids before they enter the patient. Insulating covers for IV fluid bags and the administration line are available.

Intravenous Fluids

All patients undergoing anesthesia should receive IV fluids, although they seldom do unless they are considered critical or are expected to be under anesthesia for a prolonged time. Dental patients need fluid support just as much as any surgical patient, if for no other reason than to provide IV access in the event of an emergency.

Administration of most anesthetic drugs causes vasodilatation, as discussed above. This vasodilatation results in a relative hypovolemia; the patient still has the same volume of blood it had before anesthesia (i.e., 70 ml/kg), but the expanded vasculature means that more space is available to fill. The following analogy is appropriate: A water balloon is filled with water until it is turgid. Then, air is blown into the balloon to expand it further before it is knotted. The balloon still has the same amount of water it had previously, but it is less full and taut than it was before. To counteract relative hypovolemia in dental patients (particularly older ones who may not be able to compensate), fluid must be added to fill this new void. Renal, hepatic, and cerebral perfusion may already be marginal, although compensated. Use of vasodilators without fluid support is often enough to tip the scales from compensation to decompensation, resulting in overt renal, hepatic, or cerebral dysfunction later.

Patients who are intubated or connected to anesthetic machines are particularly susceptible to dehydration. Awake patients warm and humidify inhaled gases via their nasal turbinates, but these are bypassed by the ETT. In addition, the gases from the anesthesia machine are dry. Water vapor is actually lost as it travels from the patient to the anesthetic machine. Condensation is apparent on the inspiratory or expiratory valve domes or the corrugated hoses of a circle system. When using a nonrebreathing system, none of this water vapor is recycled to the patient.

Owners are usually instructed to keep the patient from eating the evening before the procedure. (The patient is said to be "NPO.") Allowing the patient access to water up to the time of admission to the practice is ideal. However, the patient may not have consumed sufficient water during the night or in the morning because it did not get its morning meal. The owner may have misinterpreted the NPO instructions and taken water away as well as well as food; alternatively, the policy of the practice may be to prevent the patient from drinking as well as eating. Regardless of the reason, many older patients arrive at the practice mildly dehydrated.

The normal daily fluid requirement for dental patients is 70 to 90 ml/kg/day. Anesthesia, however, alters this requirement for many of the reasons already discussed. Fluid maintenance during anesthesia is generally considered to be 10 ml/kg/hr for the first hour, then 5 to 10 ml/kg/hr for subsequent hours. Of course, the exact rate of fluid administration should be adjusted based on the patient's response and physiologic parameters. Even the occasional patient that is maintained with a total intravenous anesthetic (TIVA) technique should receive IV fluids. Termination of the effects of injectable anesthetics, unlike inhalants, is via hepatic and/or renal metabolism and excretion. The provision of IV fluid support maintains normal hepatic and renal blood flow, allowing normal termination of the drugs' effects. The duration of action for many injectable drugs is often significantly longer than the procedure itself. Fluid support is therefore needed until the patient is fully recovered from the effects of injectable drugs.

Use of IV fluids requires caution. IV administration sets are available in several drop sizes. The most common ones are 15 and 60 drops/ml, although 10 and 20 drop/ml sets are also available. In patients less than 20 to 30 pounds, 60 drops/ml (also called *microdrip* or *pediatric*) sets should be used for better control of fluid flow rates. In extremely small patients (e.g., cats, toy breeds), Buretrol administration sets prevent inadvertent administration of fatal volumes of fluids. Such accidents sometimes occur after large bags of fluid are allowed to run rapidly or for long periods of time. Buretrols also make measuring and recording small volumes of fluids easier. Use of 500-ml (or smaller) fluid bags also reduces the risk of fluid overadministration in smaller patients.

PAIN MANAGEMENT

Although veterinarians decide which type of analgesics to use, technicians should understand some basic concepts of pain management. Even the least invasive dental procedure (e.g., hand scaling) has the potential to cause pain, and more invasive procedures are often quite painful. Pain has four components: transduction, transmission, modulation, and perception (Fig. 5-21). An analgesic technique blocking

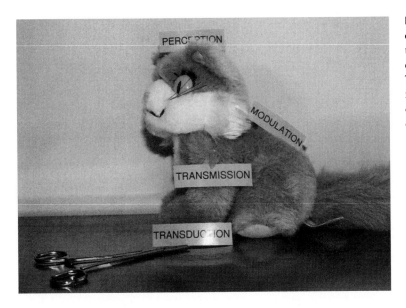

FIGURE 5-21 "Molly" demonstrating the location of the 4 modalities of pain: Transduction (at the site of injury), Transmission (peripheral nerves), Modulation (spinal cord), and Perception (cerebral cortex).

more than one component results in better and more complete analgesia than does a technique blocking only one component. The commonly used methods of providing intraoperative and postoperative analgesia for dental patients are parenteral opioids (modulation), parenteral NSAIDs (transduction), local nerve blocks (transmission), and inhalant anesthetics (perception). Doses of commonly used parenteral analgesic drugs are listed in Table 5-2.

Although detrimental to any patient, pain is a particular problem for older patients with marginally compensated organ function. Pain activates the sympathetic nervous system, resulting in the "fight or flight" response. This response is characterized by peripheral, renal, and splanchnic vasoconstriction; increased heart rate; increased resting metabolic rate; increased oxygen consumption; increased hepatic work (gluconeogenesis); and many other complications. In patients with marginal cardiac, renal, or hepatic function, the stress of pain often results in de-

---

TABLE 5-2
Common Parenteral Analgesic Drugs

Drug	Dose	Route
Morphine	0.5-1.0 mg/kg (D)	IM, IV*
	0.1-0.3 mg/kg (C)	IM, IV
Oxymorphone	0.05-0.2 mg/kg	IM, IV
Butorphanol	0.1-0.3 mg/kg	IM, IV
Hydromorphone	0.08-0.2 mg/kg (D)	IM
Meperidine	2-4 mg/kg	IM
Fentanyl	5-10 μg/kg	IM, IV
Buprenorphine	5-20 μg/kg	IM, IV
Pentazocine	1.65-3.3 mg/kg	IM, IV
Ketoprofen†	1.0-2.2 mg/kg (D)	IM, IV
Flunixin†	0.25-1.0 mg/kg (D)	
Phenylbutazone†	14-22 mg/kg, up to 800 mg per day (D)	PO, IV
	5 mg/kg (C)	PO
Carprofen†	2.2 mg/kg (D)	PO
Xylazine	0.5-1.1 mg/kg	IM, IV
Medetomidine	5-40 μg/kg (D)	IM, IV
	10-80 μg/kg	IM, IV
Ketamine	0.1-0.2 mg/kg	IV

*IV doses are generally 50% of the appropriate IM dose for that patient.
†NSAIDs are generally not recommended for use in cats.

compensation during the procedure, during recovery, or in the days immediately after the procedure.

SUMMARY

Airway management is without a doubt the most important aspect of a successful outcome to a dental procedure that requires anesthesia. Due to the very nature of the procedure, aspiration of water or foreign material is always a possibility, even with the patient in a head-down position. Because most dental patients are older, support of normal physiologic functions is necessary to ensure that patients are not harmed in the process of correcting their dental diseases. Understanding the monitors and acting on the information they provide are vital to preventing problems before a crisis develops. Supporting the patient with external heat, intravenous fluids, and analgesics helps ensure a positive outcome after the procedure is completed.

With regard to the example at the beginning of the chapter, several events during this simple procedure may have contributed to Mitzi's death. The endotracheal tube may have been too long, and during the procedure (or when Mitzi was turned) the tube may have entered a main stem bronchus, resulting in one-lung anesthesia and profound hypoxia. If this was indeed the case, during CPR the tube was still in a bronchus and the technician's attempts to revive Mitzi with 100% O_2 resulted in only one lung being ventilated.

Alternatively, the doses of "ace" or other premedicants may not have been scaled down as appropriate for a patient of Mitzi's age and temperament. Mitzi received the standard amount of an IV induction drug rather than a dosage that was titrated to effect. Mitzi was then maintained on an inhalant anesthetic at a predetermined vaporizer setting rather than a reduced setting to match the reduced anesthetic requirements of older and/or heavily premedicated patients. As a result of any one or combination of these factors, Mitzi received an overdose of potent cardiovascular depressant drugs, suffered profound vasodilatation, developed hypovolemic shock, and underwent cardiac arrest.

Complicating the situation, Mitzi did not receive intravenous fluids during the procedure. Her overly cautious owner had taken Mitzi's food and water away at 6 PM the evening before, and because Mitzi usually sleeps most of the day, she drank only at her evening meal. As a result, she was dehydrated when she arrived at the practice that morning. The drugs (sedatives, inhalant anesthetics) she received are potent vasodilators, and even though the doses were adjusted to her needs, her dehydration prevented her from compensating for the relative hypovolemia. As a result, Mitzi experienced hypovolemic shock and cardiac arrest.

Moreover, during the procedure Mitzi was soaked with a great deal of water. Dental procedures are performed at a tub table on a rack to allow the water to drain. Because this event took place during the summer, the office was air-conditioned. Because Mitzi is small, she was placed on a nonrebreathing circuit. She was on IV fluids, but either they were not warmed or her drip rate was slow enough to cause the fluid to cool to room temperature before entering her vein. Her temperature dropped rapidly during the procedure, and when she reached 80° F, her heart fibrillated. The technician realized that Mitzi had undergone cardiac arrest after turning her.

The reader is encouraged to consider other factors that may have caused Mitzi's death or, had Mitzi lived, would have created problems during the next several days to a month after the procedure. An understanding of complications and the various ways to prevent them reduces the likelihood that a patient will die during the routine use of anesthesia.

REFERENCES

West JB: *Respiratory physiology: the essentials,* ed 3, Baltimore, 1985, Williams and Wilkins.

Thurmon JC, Tranquilli WJ, Benson GJ, editors: *Lumb and Jones' veterinary anesthesia,* ed 3, Baltimore, 1996, Williams and Wilkins.

Muir WW III et al, editors: *Handbook of veterinary anesthesia,* ed 2, St Louis, 1995, Mosby.

McKelvey D, Hollingshead KW, McBride DF, editors: *Small animal anesthesia: canine and feline practice (Vol II, Mosby's fundamentals of veterinary technology),* St Louis, 1994, Mosby.

Worksheet

STUDENT NAME: _____

1. With regard to dental procedures, the following aspects of anesthesia are especially crucial. They are as follows:

   a) _____ b) _____ c) _____

   d) _____ e) _____.

2. Of the above, which is mentioned several times?

   _____.

3. The _____ and associated structures are essential for gas anesthesia.

4. The main purpose of the respiratory tract (or lungs) is to deliver _____ to the blood and eliminate _____ _____ that has been produced by the peripheral tissues.

5. Hemoglobin saturation measures the percentage of _____ that is bound with O_2, with _____% being the maximum.

6. Conducting airways include the _____, _____ and _____, _____, _____, _____, _____, and each successive branching of the bronchi down to the bronchioles.

7. When using an ultrasonic scaler, large volumes of water flood the pharyngeal area, risking _____ of water and loosened debris.

8. **All** animals undergoing dental procedures should be intubated with a _____ _____ _____ (_____ _____ _____ _____).

9. Check each cuff before induction of the patient. Gently but fully inflate each cuff, remove the syringe, and allow the cuff to remain inflated for _____ - _____ minutes.

10. Select _____ CETT sizes—one that you think will _____ the patient, one a size _____, and one a size _____.

11. _____ tube size is important because larger tubes fill the trachea more fully, reducing the risk of fluids and debris from entering the lungs should the cuff fail.

12. A commonly overlooked step is to _____ the endotracheal tube.

13. A cuff sealed to _____-_____ cm of water pressure is sufficient to prevent water from passing the cuff in a recumbent dog, with its head either level or lower than its body.

14. Packing the _____ prevents debris from entering the pharynx, larynx, and trachea cranial to the cuff and serves as a "second line of defense" should the cuff lose its seal during the procedure.

15. The initial _____ is often due to the rapidly delivered high concentration of induction drug(s) suppressing the respiratory center or lightly anesthetized patients voluntarily _____ _____ _____.

16. After _____ - _____ minutes the trachealis muscle relaxes and the internal diameter of the trachea is larger than it was at intubation.

17. The "_____ _____" is the hole in the side of the tube between the cuff and the tip.

18. The patient should **never** be moved, turned, or otherwise repositioned while _____ to the circuit.

19. Technicians should be familiar with the _____ used by the practice and should know the capabilities, limitations, and causes of false readings of each.

20. _____ patients undergoing anesthesia should receive IV fluids.

6

Pathogenesis of Periodontal Disease

Clients often ask, "Why does my pet have periodontal disease when all the pets I have had in the past had no dental problems?" Many factors determine the reason one patient develops periodontal disease and another does not (Box 6-1). These factors are as follows: age, species, breed, genetics, chewing behavior, diet, grooming habits (which can cause impaction of hair around the tooth and in the gingival sulcus), orthodontic occlusion, health status, home care, frequency of professional dental care, and bacterial flora of the oral cavity.

PERIODONTAL DISEASE

Periodontal disease is an inflammation and infection of the tissues surrounding the tooth, collectively called the *periodontium*. Periodontal disease is characterized by movement of the gingival margin toward the apex (exposing more crown and root) and migration of the attached gingiva with associated loss of the periodontal ligament and bone surrounding the tooth. An older term, *pyorrhea*, which indicates discharge of pus from the periodontium, is no longer used.

Systemic Effects of Periodontal Disease

The systemic effects of periodontal disease are fairly well documented in humans. Research in veterinary medicine is still ongoing. Theoretically, bacteria from infected tissues enter the bloodstream. Organs such as the lungs, kidney, and liver are most susceptible to infection.

Etiology

A glycoprotein component of saliva, known as the *acquired pellicle,* attaches to the tooth surface. The pellicle, which takes only 20 minutes to form, helps bacteria attach to the tooth surface. Approximately 6 to 8 hours after pellicle formation, bacteria start to colonize the tooth surface. This bacterial layer is known as *plaque.* The bacteria

---

BOX 6-1
Factors that Cause Periodontal Disease

Age	Grooming habits
Species	Orthodontic occlusion
Breed	Patient health status
Genetics	Home care
Chewing behavior	Frequency of professional care
Diet	Bacterial flora of oral cavity

---

that have colonized the tooth surface die. The bacteria that are attached to the tooth absorb calcium from saliva and become calcified. This new substance is known as *tartar* or *calculus.*

Types of Bacteria

The healthy gingival flora is made up of mostly gram-positive aerobic bacteria. These bacteria require oxygen to survive. As periodontal disease progresses, gram-negative bacteria begin to colonize the tooth surface. The aerobic bacteria metabolize oxygen, creating an environment in which the anaerobic (those that live without oxygen) bacteria start to develop. As the condition progresses, spirochetes begin to colonize. The bacteria are arranged in what is called a *biofilm,* which is an aggregate of bacterial colonies protected by a polysaccharide complex. It is the disruption of this biofilm, more than anything else, that is important in the control of periodontal disease.

Location of Plaque

Plaque is found in a number of areas around the tooth. Plaque can be supragingival. It can be subgingival in four different areas. It can be free-floating in the pocket or sulcus. It can be attached to the tooth or gingiva. Perhaps the worst plaque is the type that infiltrates the gingiva itself (Fig. 6-1).

Patient Response

As the bacteria infiltrate and colonize the sulcus or pocket and invade the gingival tissues, the patient attempts to fight the infection. *[Sulcus. A groove. In veterinary dentistry, it usually refers to the gingival sulcus present, in healthy patients with healthy gingiva, between the free gingiva and the surface of the tooth and extending around the tooth's circumference.]* White blood cells produce antibodies and send chemical signals into the system to stimulate other cells to come in and attack the bacteria. The bacteria often contain endotoxins (sometimes called *lipopolysaccharides,* or *LPS*) and enzymes that are toxic to the gingival tissues.

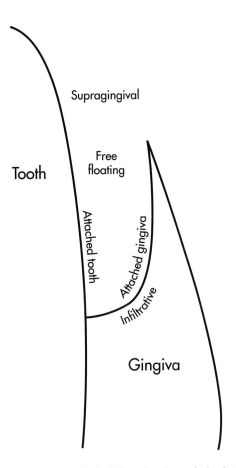

FIGURE 6-1 Types of plaque: supragingival, free-floating subgingival, attached to tooth or gingiva, invasive into gingiva.

Pathogenesis

As the inflammation continues, the gingiva loosens from the tooth. As a result, the gingiva separates from the tooth and a space between the tooth and gingiva develops. This space is known as the *pocket.* Deeper in the periodontium, loss of tissue and bone support indicates the beginning of the disease. If the patient is not treated and the disease is allowed to progress, deeper pockets form.

Without the gingival epithelial attachment, the gingiva begins to recede. *[Epithelial attachment. The epithelium attaching the gingiva to the tooth.]* In multirooted teeth, the furcation (the area at which the roots join the crown) begins to be exposed. Furcation exposure is classified by depth (Box 6-2). Class 1 furcation exposure is less than 1 mm; Class 2 exposure is greater than 1 mm but not fully through; Class 3 is complete furcation exposure. As bone loss proceeds, the tooth may become mobile. Finally, if the loss of attachment is sufficient, the tooth may fall out.

BOX 6-2
Classes of Furcation Exposure

Class 1 furcation Exposure less than 1mm	**Class 3 furcation** Complete furcation Probe able to pass through furcation
Class 2 furcation Exposure greater than 1 mm Not fully through	

Initial Signs

Most commonly, clients report halitosis (bad breath) as the patient's periodontal disease progresses. This is often mistakenly called "doggy breath." This condition, however, is not normal. It is caused by periodontal disease and is one of the first signs of this condition. Clients may report that their pets are not eating well. Occasionally, patients drool, and blood may be noted in the saliva. Clients may also observe the patient pawing at its mouth.

Upon oral examination, red, inflamed gingiva may be noted. The gingiva may bleed easily when probed (Fig. 6-2). Fragile capillaries in the inflamed tissue cause this bleeding. An accumulation of plaque and calculus is evident. However, it is important to note that the amount of plaque and calculus does not always correspond to the degree of periodontal disease present.

Staging Periodontal Disease

As an aid to treatment, the degree of periodontal disease is staged. If the patient is cooperative, a general evaluation of the periodontal stage, based on factors such as plaque, calculus, inflammation, and topography, may be performed while the patient is awake. However, general anesthesia is necessary for a more complete evaluation, which includes a periodontal probe and intraoral radiographic procedures. The classification system used here progresses from Stage 1 through Stage 4. The patient's worst tooth is used to establish the stage of periodontal disease. Consequently, even if the rest of the teeth are healthy, the patient is said to have Stage 4 periodontal disease if the worst tooth is at this stage. In reality, each tooth must be evaluated and charted for effective treatment.

Healthy Gingiva

Healthy gingiva has a knifelike margin and is coral pink or a pigmented color (Fig. 6-3). Smooth gingival topography must be noted. The term *topography* refers to the surface features of the gingiva as it flows from tooth to tooth. Generally, as periodontal disease progresses, the surface features become irregular and the even flow from tooth to tooth is lost. Healthy gingival tissue is firm. Close observation reveals

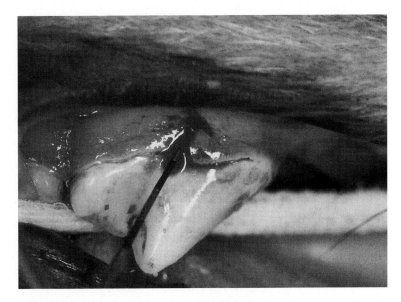

FIGURE 6-2 Bleeding of gingiva caused by light probing with a periodontal probe.

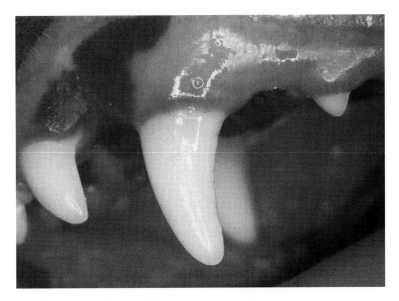

FIGURE 6-3 Healthy gingiva.

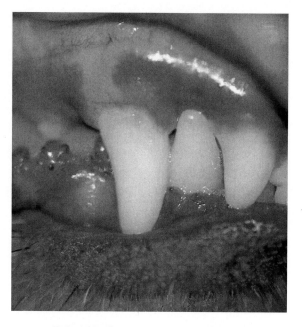

FIGURE 6-4 Stage 1: early gingivitis.

the presence of blood vessels at the gingival margins; this is known as *defined stippling. [Free gingival margin. The unattached edge of the gingiva that lies against the tooth surface.]* With use of a periodontal probe the normal minimal sulcular depth is 2 to 3 mm in dogs and 0.5 to 1 mm in cats. Evidence of previous disease may be present but does not necessarily appear.

Early Gingivitis

Redness of the gingiva at the crest and a mild amount of plaque are noted in the early stage of gingivitis (Fig. 6-4). The fine blood vessels at the gingival margins are more difficult to visualize. Radiographically, little noticeable change from early gingivitis is apparent. Early gingivitis is reversible with treatment. Stage 1 gingivitis may appear 2 to 4 days after plaque accumulation in previously healthy gingiva and is localized to the gingival sulcus, which includes the junctional epithelium and the most coronal part of the connective tissue.

Advanced Gingivitis

Advanced gingivitis is similar to the early stage in that it is still reversible, although an increase in inflammation, including edema and development of subgingival plaque, is apparent (Fig. 6-5). The amount of supragingival plaque and calculus is also increased. The gingival topography has started to become irregular but is still in satisfactory condition. Root exposure has not yet occurred. Radiographs exhibit little noticeable change. Plaque-induced gingivitis can be reversed with the initiation of plaque-control measures (e.g., dental scaling and prophylaxis, home care).

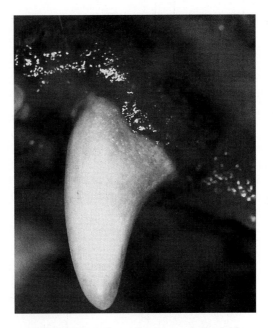

FIGURE 6-5 Stage 2: advanced gingivitis.

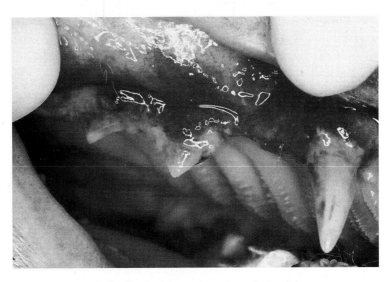

FIGURE 6-6 Stage 3: early periodontitis.

Early Periodontitis

Early periodontitis includes a moderate loss of attachment or moderate pocket formation with a 10% to 30% loss of bone support (Fig. 6-6). Furcation exposure, inadequate gingival topography, recession, and hypertrophy may be present. *[Furcation. The space between tooth roots where the roots join the crown.]* Tooth mobility may also be observed in some cases. The gingiva bleeds with gentle probing at this stage. Radiographs may show subgingival calculus, and a rounding of the alveolar crestal bone at the cervical portion of the tooth can be seen upon careful examination. *[**Alveolar crest.** The most coronal ridge of bone between two adjacent teeth or between the roots of a tooth.]*

Established Periodontitis

In established periodontitis the teeth show advanced breakdown of the support tissues, with severe pocket depth or severe recession of the gingiva (Fig. 6-7). Some of the signs that may be associated with Stage 4, or advanced periodontal disease, are severe inflammation, deep pocket formation, gingival recession, bone loss, pus, and mobility. The gingiva usually bleeds easily when probed. A loss of gingival topography is apparent. Radiographs show subgingival calculus and bone loss.

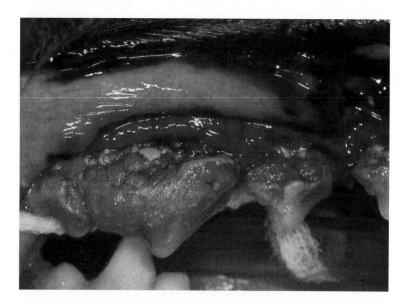

FIGURE 6-7 Stage 4: established periodontitis.

Worksheet

STUDENT NAME: _____

1. Periodontal disease is an _____ and _____ of the tissues surrounding the tooth. It is characterized by movement of the gingiva toward the apex and migration of the junctional epithelium with associated loss of the periodontal ligament and bone surrounding the tooth.

2. A glycoprotein component of saliva, known as the _____ _____, attaches to the tooth surface.

3. As periodontal disease progresses, _____ _____ bacteria begin to colonize.

4. Subgingival plaque may be found in what four areas? _____, _____, _____, _____.

5. _____ _____ is not normal.

6. The amount of _____ and _____ may not always correspond to the degree of periodontal disease that is present.

7. Healthy gingiva has a _____ _____ and is coral pink or a pigmented color.

8. Stage 1 can appear _____ to _____ days after plaque accumulation in previously healthy gingiva.

9. Stage 2 is known as _____ _____.

10. The stage with advanced breakdown, severe pocket depth, bleeding easily on probing, pus, bone loss, and mobility is Stage _____.

7

The Complete Prophy

Veterinarians and technicians often speak of performing a "prophy" or "dental." This usage is incorrect and may often mislead the client with regard to the patient's true condition. Because the word *prophylaxis,* which means prevention of or protective treatment for disease, is sometimes confused with "prophylactic," or "condom," the dental profession shortened the word to *prophy.* The difference between performing a prophy and periodontal therapy is extremely important. The term *prophy* is often used incorrectly to indicate the treatment of periodontal disease rather than its prevention. This important distinction must be kept in mind when discussing treatment plans with the client. One analogy is to compare a prophy with a vaccination for a disease rather than the treatment for that disease. Once the patient has periodontal disease, far more extensive treatment is required. In this case the clinician should discuss with the client the necessary steps and options (which may include extractions) to treat the condition. A complete prophy requires several important instruments and pieces of equipment (Box 7-1).

PREPARATION FOR THE PROCEDURE

Before performing the prophy, the veterinarian should discuss the procedure with the client and provide a written estimate of its cost. After obtaining the client's consent, the veterinarian should develop a contingency plan in case additional problems are discovered under anesthesia and the client must be contacted. The client should provide instructions so that the veterinary staff knows how to proceed in case the client is unavailable during the procedure. Options include the following:
1. Proceed with recommended procedures.
2. Attempt to call first; if the client cannot be reached, proceed with recommended procedures.
3. Do nothing if the client cannot be contacted.

Consideration should also be given to preoperative blood profiles, intravenous fluids, preoperative antibiotics (if indicated), anesthetic protocol (including preoperative agents, induction, anesthesia, and patient monitoring). Inhalation anesthesia with an endotracheal tube is necessary to prevent the aspiration of fluids, dental calculus, and other debris.

BOX 7-1

Instruments and Equipment Needed for the Complete Prophy

Sickle scaler: H6/7, S6/7, N6/7, SH6/7, or Cislak P-12
Curette: Barnhardt 5/6, Columbia 13/14, or Cislak P-10
Calculus-removing forceps
Periodontal probe/explorer: double-ended, Williams type with 1-mm markers (sizes go up to 15 mm [Hu-Friedy] or 18 mm [Cislak])
#2 Pigtail explorer
Ultrasonic or sonic scaler
Low-speed handpiece
Prophy angle
Prophy cup
Prophy paste
Sharpening stones
Disclosing solution
Chlorhexidine rinse

ANESTHESIA INDUCTION

After anesthesia is induced (see Chapter 5), the patient is intubated and stabilized. An overview of the oral cavity should take place to establish that the initial diagnosis (Stage 1 or Stage 2 periodontal disease) was correct and revision of the treatment plan is not necessary.

STEPS TO THE COMPLETE PROPHY

The complete prophy entails several steps (Box 7-2). According to the general sequence, the oral cavity is generally evaluated, large pieces of calculus are removed, and the periodontal area is probed for pocket depth and the presence of subgingival calculus. Next, the subgingival calculus is removed, and the teeth are evaluated to ensure that they and the entire periodontal area are completely clean. Then, the degree of disease is evaluated, and further diagnostic tests are performed. Any pathologic condition of the oral cavity should be noted and charted. Home-care instruction should be given to the client either before (to assess compliance) or after the procedure.

When to Use Antibiotics?

Ultimately, the decision to administer antibiotics is the veterinarian's. The veterinarian evaluates the patient and prescribes antibiotics if indicated. Generally, antibiotics are not necessary for healthy patients with Stage 1 and Stage 2 periodontal

---

BOX 7-2
Steps to the Complete Prophy

1. Preliminary examination and evaluation
2. Gross calculus removal
3. Periodontal probing (and periodontal charting)
4. Subgingival calculus removal
5. Missed plaque/calculus detection
6. Polishing
7. Sulcus irrigation
8. Periodontal diagnostics
9. Final charting
10. Home care

disease. Antibiotics are indicated for Stages 3 and 4 and patients who are compromised by health conditions (e.g., disease of the liver, kidney, or heart) or viral infections (e.g., feline leukemia virus or feline immunodeficiency virus).

Patient Care

Once anesthetized, the patient should be positioned in lateral recumbency on a grate over a table sink or on a specially designed dental table that allows the fluids used in the dental procedure to drain. Mouth gags should not be used for more than a few minutes; when they are used, care should be taken not to overextend the mandible. Overextension of the mandible may lead to stretching and tearing of the ligaments and muscles of the jaw. Instead, the mouth should be propped open with the nonworking hand (Fig. 7-1).

Step 1: Preliminary Examination and Evaluation

Ideally the patient has allowed the practitioner to perform a preliminary examination of the oral cavity before induction of anesthesia. However, some patients may not allow this examination at all or, at best, only for a brief time. Therefore the first step in a prophy is a more complete evaluation to evaluate the necessary diagnostic and treatment measures.

Step 2: Supragingival Gross Calculus Removal

The next step of the procedure is to remove supragingival gross calculus. Many types of instruments may be used to perform this step.

Hand scalers

Hand scalers are used for supragingival removal of calculus. They should not be inserted below the gumline. Scalers are particularly effective in removing calculus from

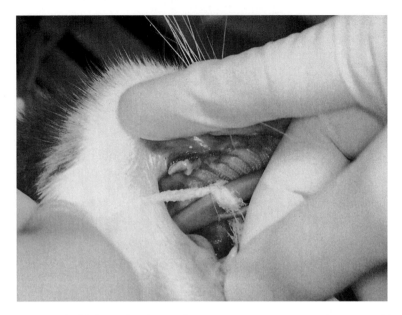

FIGURE 7-1 To hold the patient's mouth open, operators may use the nonworking hand. Here, the index finger is used to lift the upper lip while the middle finger opens the jaw.

the developmental groove of the fourth premolar. A pull stroke (a stroke pulling the calculus toward the coronal aspect) is used to remove calculus.

Calculus removal forceps

Use of calculus removal forceps is a fairly quick method for removing supragingival calculus. The longer tip is placed over the crown, the shorter under the calculus. The calculus is cleaved off when the tips are brought together (Fig. 7-2). When using calculus removal forceps, the operator should be extremely careful not to damage the gingiva or create an iatrogenic slab fracture.

Ultrasonic or sonic scalers

Ultrasonic or sonic scalers are used to quickly remove the smaller deposits of supragingival calculus. Ultrasonic scalers vibrate in the range of 18,000 to 45,000 cycles per second. When properly applied, this vibration breaks up or pulverizes calculus on the surface of teeth. Because ultrasonic instruments can damage teeth by mechanical etching or thermal heating, they should be used with caution (Fig. 7-3). For supragingival scaling, use of the side of a beaver tail tip is preferable rather than the end of the tip. This section of the chapter discusses supragingival scaling, but the same principles apply to the use of ultrasonic or sonic scalers in subgingival scaling. Often, supragingival and subgingival scaling are performed at the same time.

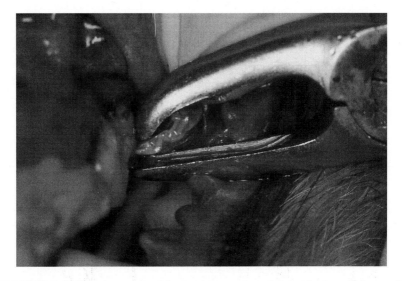

FIGURE 7-2 Calculus removal forceps are used to cleave calculus off the tooth.

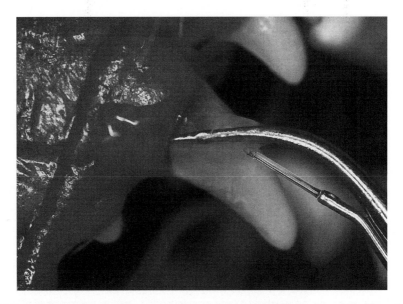

FIGURE 7-3 Ultrasonic scalers are used to remove calculus from the tooth. Note the adequate water flow, which prevents overheating of the tooth.

Power instrument grasp

The ultrasonic instrument should be grasped lightly, not tightly. It should feel balanced in the hand, with minimal pull from the handpiece cord. The handpiece, not the hands, must be allowed to do the work (Fig. 7-4). The handpiece is balanced on the index or middle finger. A modified pen grasp is not as important in holding the ultrasonic or sonic scaler as it is with hand instruments (Fig. 7-5). To decrease stress on the hand from the pull on the handpiece cord, the cord may be looped over the little finger (Fig. 7-6). As opposed to hand instruments, in which a fulcrum is used to provide leverage for the pulling stroke, ultrasonic scalers do not require a fulcrum. The hand is used as a guide for the ultrasonic handpiece.

Water flow

Water flow is required to prevent overheating of the teeth and damage to the pulp. With the broad-based, beaver-type inserts, an ample supply of water is necessary for irrigation (Fig. 7-7). Less water is required to cool the smaller tips. The water flow can be adjusted to a smaller halo, almost a drip, just enough to cool the tip (Fig. 7-8).

Insertion

Turning on the handpiece before insertion provides a water supply and thereby eases the insertion of the tip in the sulcus, should subgingival scaling be performed at the same time as supragingival scaling.

Pressure

The operator should use a light touch, keeping the tip moving while traveling around the circumference of the tooth and not stopping in any area.

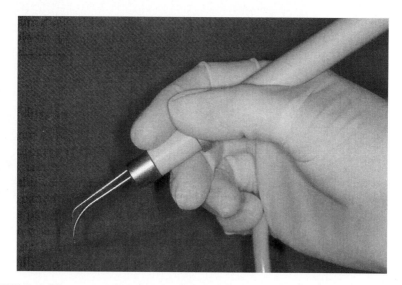

FIGURE 7-4 The operator's hand should assume a passive role in holding the ultrasonic scaler.

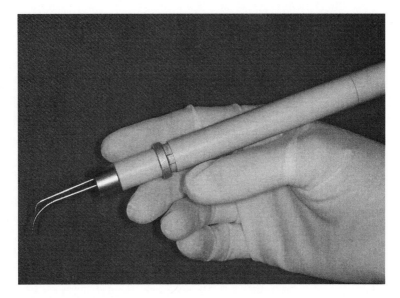

FIGURE 7-5 The handpiece is resting on the hand rather than being grasped by it.

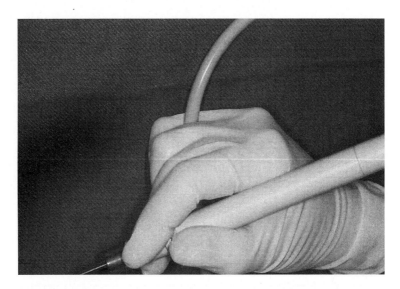

FIGURE 7-6 The handpiece cord can be looped over the little finger to prevent "back drag."

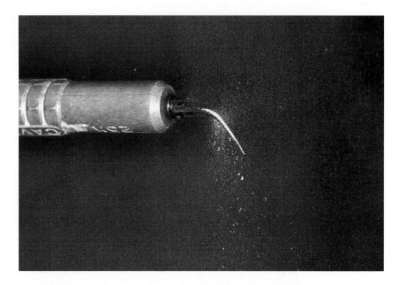

FIGURE 7-7 A greater water supply is necessary for broad-based tips.

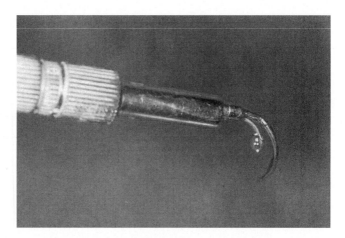

FIGURE 7-8 Only a drip is required for the thinner subgingival handpieces.

Adaptation

Unlike hand instruments, ultrasonic and sonic instruments do not need cutting edges. However, the tip motion of the instrument must be understood to take advantage of the maximal cleaning stroke. The side of the tip should be held parallel to the tooth surface. The tip of the ultrasonic instrument should not be pointed at the tooth surface or held at a 90-degree angle to the tooth. Doing so could damage the tooth surface by heating up the pulp; it also provides less cleaning surface and therefore is less effective (Fig. 7-9). The instrument tip is kept parallel with the long axis of the tooth. A straight shank can be used when working straight down the tooth (Fig. 7-10). A curved shank will allow working around a crown or in a furcation (Fig. 7-11).

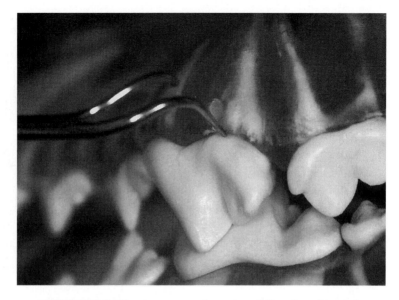

FIGURE 7-9 The tip must not be pointed directly at the tooth.

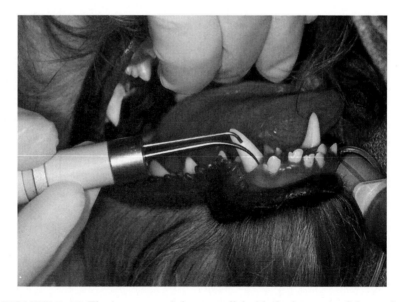

FIGURE 7-10 The instrument is kept parallel with the long axis of the tooth.

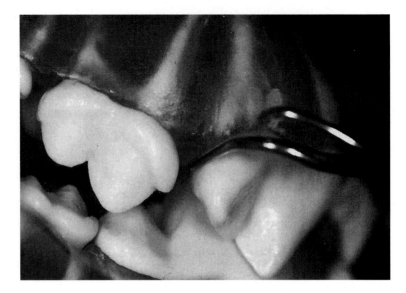

FIGURE 7-11 A furcation tip can be used to work around a crown or into a furcation.

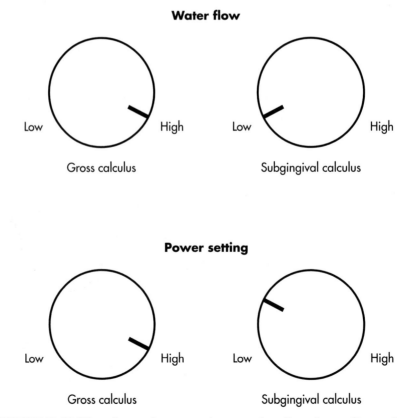

FIGURE 7-12 Water flow and power settings must be adjusted according to the use.

BOX 7-3
Ultrasonic Technique (Remember DENTAL)

Digits
- An extraoral finger rest is useful for maxillary posterior teeth.
- Fingers should rest on the teeth for maxillary anterior and mandibular areas.
- A stable fulcrum is not always necessary.

Engage
- Activate the tip of the instrument and direct the tip subgingivally.
- Water lavage will facilitate a comfortable entry into the sulcus.

Neutral
- Use a balanced instrument grasp; the instrument should feel balanced in the hand with no pull from the cord.
- Use a light pen or modified pen grasp.

Technique
- Brush away the calculus, using sweeping cross strokes.

Adaptation
- Unlike curettes, which have a specific cutting edge, ultrasonic and sonic instruments are active on at least 2 sides when in contact with the tooth surface.
- The side of the tip is held parallel to the tooth surface.
- The end of the tip should not be adapted to the tooth surface at a 90 degree angle.

Light touch
- Apply extremely light pressure, equivalent to that used when blanching the tissue on the back of the hand.

Ultrasonic technique

The ultrasonic technique includes the following steps:
- Start out with sweeping cross strokes.
- Next, work in various directions (i.e., coronal apical, oblique, circumferential).
- To reach furcations, use oblique or corkscrew tips. Different tips have been created to reach different difficult areas.
- Avoid pressing the scaler tip on the tooth surface too hard; excessive force can result in thermal damage and render the equipment tip ineffective because it dampens the vibrations.

Power settings

Higher power settings should be used for the broad, beaver-tail–type tips. The power should be decreased to lower settings when thin subgingival tips are used. Failure to decrease the power may cause fracturing of the tip or render it ineffective because tips are manufactured to operate in optimal frequency ranges (Fig. 7-12; Box 7-3).

Rotary scalers

Since its introduction to veterinary medicine, the rotary scaler has been very controversial. Its acceptance in human dentistry has been limited because the rotary scaler can easily damage teeth and requires a great deal of training and practice for safe use. Rather than scaling the teeth, this bur frequently ends up burnishing the calculus. Ineffective removal or burnishing of calculus can lead to a periodontal abscess. Veterinarians who insist on using rotary scalers should discuss them with their own dentists and hygienists. Before using the rotary scaler on their patients' teeth, veterinarians should undergo the experience first (assuming their dentists are willing).

Step 3: Periodontal Probing (and Periodontal Charting)

Probing technique

A periodontal probe should be used to measure the depth of the sulcus or pocket. Caution is necessary when applying the periodontal probe. A healthy sulcus will bleed if more than 20 grams of pressure is applied to the probe. If too much pressure is applied, the probe can puncture the junctional epithelium. The probe should be held parallel to the long axis of the tooth for an accurate reading (Fig. 7-13). Holding the probe at an angle results in an inaccurate measurement. The measured depth must be carefully evaluated when using a periodontal probe. The measurement of sulcular or pocket depth is not the same as that of attachment loss. If the marginal gingiva is at the normal cementoenamel junction, the probed depth will cor-

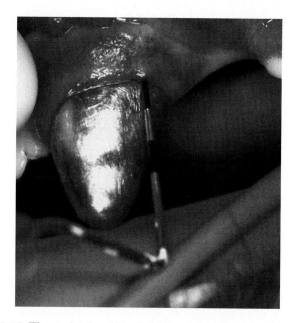

FIGURE 7-13 The probe should be held parallel to the long axis of the tooth.

respond to attachment loss. *[Cementoenamel junction. The junction at the neck of the tooth where the enamel and the cementum meet.]*

If previous recession of gingiva has occurred and the marginal gingiva has moved apically, the pocket depth will be less than the actual loss of attached gingiva. If gingival hyperplasia and a pseudopocket are present as a result, the probed depth will be greater than the actual attachment loss.

Charting

Record keeping is an important part of the dental procedure. Dental charts or stick-on labels are used for dental charting and record keeping. Because periodontal disease is progressive, charting is an important aid for follow-up visits. Accurate records establish a baseline: Subsequent measurements of the pockets, furcation exposure, and mobility are compared at each appointment, which is useful in evaluating treatment and client compliance.

The method used to chart teeth should be consistent (Fig. 7-14). The following starting order is recommended: buccal of right posterior maxilla, lingual of right posterior maxilla, lingual of right posterior mandible, and buccal of right posterior mandible. From the starting point the probing is conducted to the opposite side. Dental abnormalities, such as missing or fractured teeth, are noted. Points on each side should be measured while charting the sulcular/pocket depth. The distal, mid-

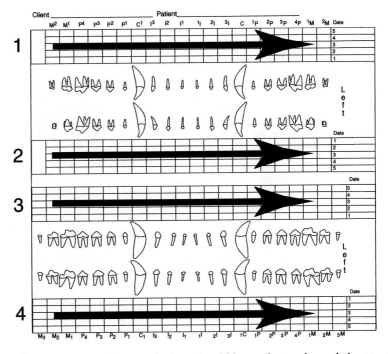

FIGURE 7-14 A consistent technique should be used to probe and chart teeth.

section, and mesial portions of the tooth are measured. One easy, quick method to chart teeth is to record the measurements with a tape recorder. This technique allows continuous measurement, and the tape can be played back later when documenting the information in the chart.

Step 4: Subgingival Calculus Removal

A curette or select ultrasonic scaler should be used to remove the calculus below the gumline. Ultrasonic scalers with subgingival tips can be used to scale and remove calculus below the gumline. Several companies make specialized inserts that can be used subgingivally. Removal of subgingival calculus is an extremely important part of the procedure. If subgingival calculus remains, the patient will not receive long-term benefits from treatment and bacterial plaque will continue destroying the periodontium, leading first to bone deterioration and eventually to tooth loss.

Hand instrument technique

The modified pen grasp is the preferred method for holding hand instruments (Fig. 7-15). In contrast to the pen grasp, in which the working end of the instrument ends up on the back side of the hand, with the modified pen grasp the working end is on the palm side. The use of a fulcrum and pull stroke results in removal of calculus.

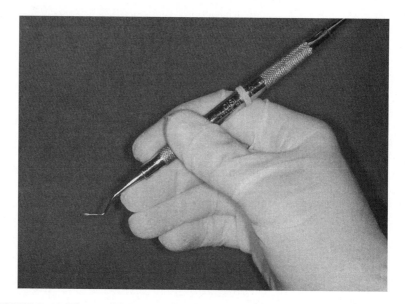

FIGURE 7-15 The modified pen grip should be used for holding hand instruments.

Modified pen grasp

The thumb and forefinger are placed at the junction of the handle and the shank of the instrument. The index finger is placed on the shank. The ring finger is held straight and placed on the surface closest to the tooth being worked on. The position of the fingers creates a "triangle of forces" that provides stability and control when the wrist-rocking motion is initiated. The middle finger, ring finger, or index finger is placed on the tooth to be scaled or an adjacent tooth. The closer the fulcrum is to the tooth being scaled, the more effective the working stroke, as a result of its greater power. This grip can be practiced by holding a pencil and drawing a small circle by rotating only on the fulcrum (ring finger) and moving the wrist. The fingers should not flex at all during this motion.

Adapting to the tooth

The curette is adapted to the tooth root surface (Fig. 7-16). If the instrument does not fit the curvature of the tooth, the opposite end of the instrument is adapted (Fig. 7-17).

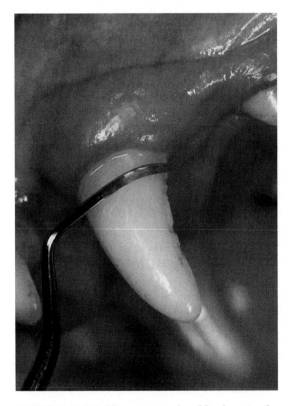

FIGURE 7-16 The curette should adapt to the tooth surface; if it does not, the opposite end should be used.

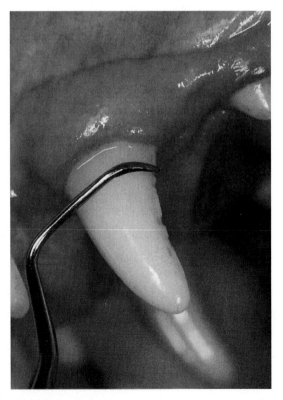

FIGURE 7-17 Proper adaptation to the tooth surface.

As the curette is inserted into the pocket, the face of the instrument should face the root surface. This is called the *closed position*. The instrument is moved over the calculus and then repositioned so that the cutting surface is under the calculus ledge. This is called the *open position*. With a rocking pull or oblique stroke, calculus is cleaved from the root surface.

Step 5: Detection of Missed Plaque and Calculus

An explorer is used to evaluate the tooth surface while checking for subgingival calculus. The tooth is inspected for missed plaque and calculus by the application of disclosing solution or by air drying, which makes the deposits appear chalky white.

Application of disclosing solution

Do you remember the dental hygienist who came to your class in elementary school to demonstrate proper tooth brushing? In such demonstrations, the hygienist gives the students disclosing tablets to chew after brushing their teeth. After rinsing their mouths, the students can see plaque they missed while brushing, which shows up brightly pigmented. Similarly, disclosing solution can be used to maintain quality control of the teeth-cleaning procedure. Painting a small amount of disclosing solution on the teeth with a cotton-tipped applicator allows detection of plaque and calculus that were missed while scaling (Fig. 7-18). After being rinsed with water, areas where plaque remains assume a red or blue pigment, depending on the brand (Fig. 7-19). Clean teeth do not retain the stain. Care should be exercised when using disclosing solution because it can stain hair and clothing.

Air-drying

Another technique to detect plaque and calculus is to dry the tooth with compressed air. Plaque and calculus appear chalky white when dry (Fig. 7-20). This technique should not be used if the integrity of the periodontium is in question because air could be blown into tissues, resulting in air being trapped in the subcutaneous tissues or possibly entering the bloodstream.

Step 6: Polishing

Polishing with an electrical or air-powered polisher removes any plaque that may have been missed and smooths the tooth surface. Because polishing generates considerable heat, a liberal amount of prophy paste should be used and only a brief period of time should be spent on each tooth (Fig. 7-21). Some researchers have expressed concern that excessive polishing could cause enamel loss. Risk of enamel loss may be a factor with humans, whose teeth may be polished 3 or 4 times a year for many years; however, most veterinary patients are lucky to have their teeth cleaned 10 times over the course of their lives.

Prophy angles are attachments on slow-speed or electric-motor handpieces that are used to polish teeth. Either screw-on types or pop-on rubber cups can be used with the prophy angle. Prophy angles come in nonreusable plastic models,

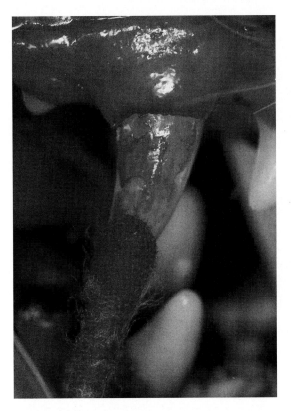

FIGURE 7-18 Disclosing solution is applied with a cotton-tipped applicator.

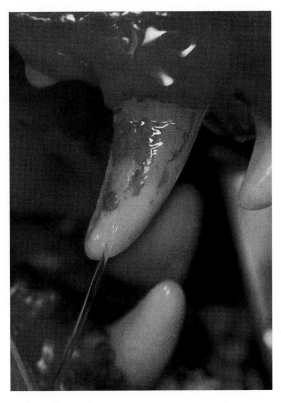

FIGURE 7-19 Water is used to irrigate the tooth. The disclosing solution stains plaque and calculus for easier observation.

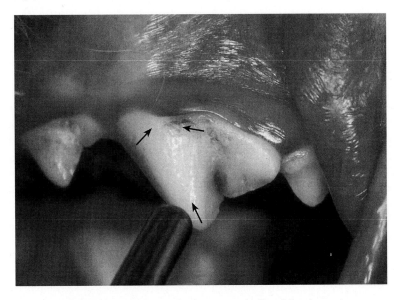

FIGURE 7-20 Dry calculus turns chalky white *(arrows)*.

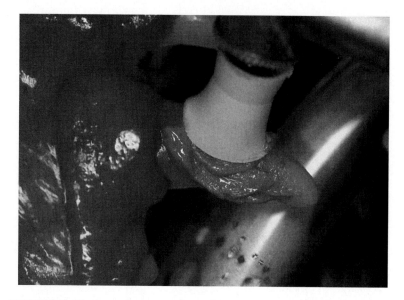

FIGURE 7-21 A prophy cup and prophy paste are used to polish the teeth.

inexpensive nonrepairable versions, and expensive nonlubricating sealed units (Fig. 7-22).

One advantage with disposable plastic prophy angles is that they are relatively inexpensive and do not need to be cleaned after use; they are simply discarded. They should not be cleaned and used on multiple patients. The rubber in the prophy cup cannot withstand multiple uses. The phrase *prophy cup* has multiple meanings. In this text a prophy cup is the rubber cup used on the prophy angle for polishing teeth, and a prophy paste holder is the cup used to hold prophy paste.

Another option is the metal, fairly inexpensive, nonrepairable prophy angle units, which must be disinfected between uses. Most require lubrication, as discussed in the equipment section.

Sealed nonrotary prophy angles are also available. They oscillate back and forth at 90 degrees. Because they do not rotate 360 degrees, they will not wrap hair around the prophy cup, which is an advantage. However, they are more expensive than other prophy angles and must be set for fewer revolutions per minute than standard prophy angles. Like the other reusable prophy angles, they must be disinfected between uses.

The most economical (but messiest) means of making prophy paste is to mix flour pumice with a slight amount of water. Many different brands of fine commercial prophy paste are available, in many different flavors. Most contain fluoride, which should not be substituted for the final irrigation. Prophy paste helps to reduce the heat that is generated while polishing. Fine paste is used to smooth down the tooth surface. Coarse paste is used to remove stains and should be followed up with fine prophy paste.

Before the teeth are polished, prophy paste is transferred from the prophy paste holder to the teeth with the prophy cup. A small amount is placed on each tooth in

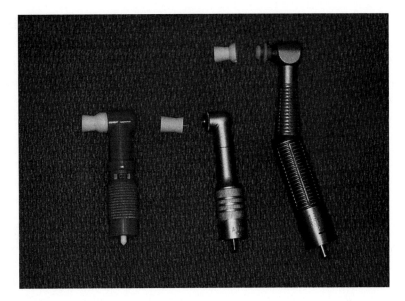

FIGURE 7-22 Plastic, metal, and oscillating prophy angles *(left to right)*.

a quadrant before turning on the unit. The teeth are polished with a low-speed handpiece at approximately 3000 to 8000 RPM. The prophy cup must be kept moving and should never linger over one area. A slight flare of the prophy cup is used to polish teeth subgingivally.

Step 7: Sulcus Irrigation and Fluoride Treatment

Gentle irrigation of the sulcus flushes out trapped debris and oxygenates the intrasulcular fluids. A saline, stannous fluoride or diluted chlorhexidine solution may be used. A blunted 23-gauge irrigation needle with syringe is effective for this. The full-strength disinfectant chlorhexidine commonly found in veterinary hospitals should never be used as a disinfectant without proper dilution. A fluoride foam may be applied to slow the reattachment of plaque after the prophy. Flurofom® is applied with a cotton-tipped applicator and allowed to sit on the tooth surface for 3 to 5 minutes (Fig. 7-23). It is then wiped (not washed) from the tooth surface.

Step 8: Periodontal Diagnostics

Diagnostics should always include periodontal probing (if not already performed) and intraoral radiology as indicated.

Periodontal radiographs

Radiographs should be taken to evaluate the dental and bony structures for periodontal bone loss, root canal disease, and other conditions (Fig. 7-24).

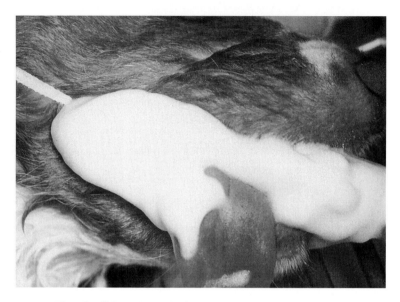

FIGURE 7-23 Flurofom® foam is applied to the tooth surface and allowed to soak for 3 to 5 minutes before it is wiped clean.

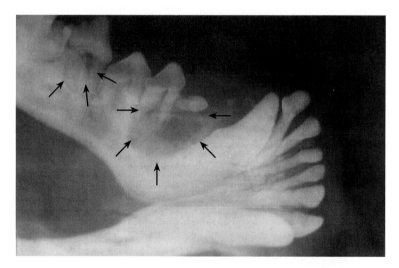

FIGURE 7-24 This radiograph demonstrates bone loss *(arrows)*.

Step 9: Final Charting

Final charting involves a review of the previously performed diagnostic and periodontal charting. This final review should include any additional treatment performed.

Step 10: Home Care

The last step in the complete prophy is home-care instruction. This subject is discussed in detail in Chapter 8.

Worksheet

STUDENT NAME: _____

1. _____ are performed for patients with healthy, Stage 1 or Stage 2 periodontal disease. _____ _____ is performed for patients with Stage 3 or Stage 4 periodontal disease.

2. The second step of the procedure is to remove supragingival _____ calculus.

3. Use of _____ _____ _____ is a fairly quick method of removing supragingival calculus.

4. Ultrasonic instruments can damage teeth by _____ _____ or _____ _____.

5. The ultrasonic instrument should be grasped _____, not _____.

6. _____ _____ is required to prevent overheating of the teeth and damage to the pulp.

7. The operator should use a _____ touch, keeping the tip moving while traveling around the circumference of the tooth and not stopping in any area.

8. The _____ pen grasp is the method of holding dental instruments.

9. Gentle irrigation of the sulcus flushes out trapped debris and _____ the intrasulcular fluids.

10. _____ should be taken to evaluate the dental and bony structures for periodontal bone loss, root canal disease, and other conditions.

8

Home-Care Instruction

Client education should begin before the procedure is performed. In addition to informing the client about the procedure, client education is an important way to evaluate the client's willingness to perform home care and the patient's willingness to accept it. The decision to save a tooth or extract it depends on the client's desire and ability to comply with home-care instructions.

CLIENT EDUCATION

All members of the veterinary office staff play important roles in the promotion of pet oral health by home-care instruction. These efforts help bond the client to the practice. Staff members should review brushing and home-care techniques with clients. If possible, a "demonstrator" dog (or cat) should be used (Fig. 8-1). Otherwise, plastic or plaster dental models can be used to show brushing techniques. These models show pathologic as well as healthy conditions. However, skulls should not be used for demonstration because some clients respond negatively to them.

Demonstration

A circular or oval motion with emphasis on the coronal direction, away from the gumline, is recommended. Staff members who are properly trained in this area foster client rapport and increase the likelihood of successful therapy. Clients should be encouraged to return for further instruction as often as necessary.

Tips for difficult cases

For patients that resist attempts to brush, flavored material or toothpaste can be placed on the toothbrush. The patient is allowed to lick the brush, with no effort made to brush the teeth or restrain the patient in any way (Fig. 8-2). Once the patient begins to become comfortable with the process, the client can begin to swipe at the teeth. Eventually, full brushing can take place. Cats may respond positively to liquid drained out of water-packed tuna.

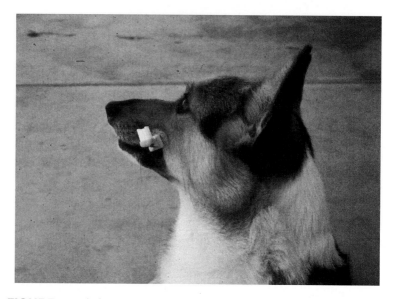

FIGURE 8-1 A demonstrator dog or cat may be used in client education.

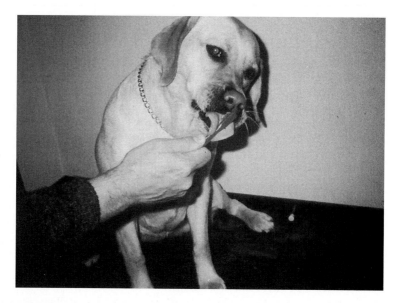

FIGURE 8-2 Simply allowing the pet to lick the brush is the first step to establishing home care.

Advanced techniques

Once the patient is accustomed to having its teeth brushed, a Dentabone®, Nylabone®, or other prop may be placed in the mouth (Fig. 8-3). The mouth is held closed, and the teeth are brushed. When the Dentabone® is used, the patient can eat the prop as a reward.

Visual Aids

Visual aids and client handouts are also beneficial in reinforcing the need for brushing and home care. Many manufacturers offer professionally designed handouts. Many clients feel reassured when they read or hear the same information from a variety of sources. Handouts are best displayed in the reception or exam rooms. Some commercial handouts leave spaces for the inclusion of the practice's name and phone number. The practitioner can also customize a handout specifically for the practice. Photographs of the dental area and equipment may increase client awareness of veterinary dentistry procedures performed in the hospital or clinic.

With the advent of computers, handouts can be customized to reflect each patient's specific condition. For example, a client whose pet has Stage 1 periodontal disease requires different educational materials than a client whose pet has Stage 4. These handouts can be linked to either diagnostic codes or service codes so that when a particular procedure is performed, the handout is generated automatically. Preprinted or computer-generated handouts provide information about periodontics, endodontics, orthodontics, and other dental diseases and treatments. Several companies make flip or wall charts that demonstrate various aspects of veterinary dentistry. Polaroid or digital photographs can be used to demonstrate each patient's

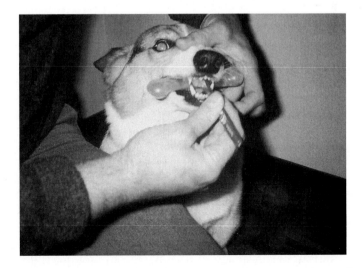

FIGURE 8-3 Once tooth brushing is accepted, a mouth prop can be used to keep the mouth open while the teeth are brushed.

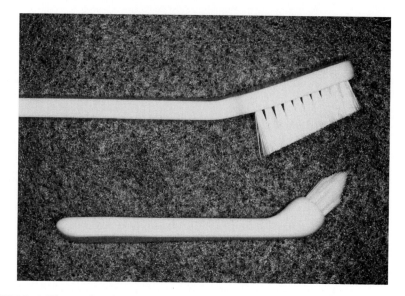

FIGURE 8-4 The top brush is the canine brush, and the bottom brush is a feline brush invented by Peter Emily, DDS, Honorary Diplomate, American Veterinary Dental College; both brushes are manufactured by Virbac®.

pathologic condition and often are a key to client communication. Videotapes showing dental procedures are also available.

PLAQUE CONTROL AND HOME CARE

Brushing Devices

The most important strategy in the prevention of periodontal disease is plaque control. There are two major methods of plaque control: mechanical and chemical. The mechanical removal of plaque is particularly important in the control of periodontal disease. Many types of devices can be used. The use of a soft, child-size or preschool toothbrush is the most effective method. Virbac (C.E.T.) makes a rubber finger toothbrush and canine and feline toothbrushes (Fig. 8-4). A cotton-tipped applicator may be effective for some patients. Smaller brushes useful for brushing the interproximal and furcation areas are available at human pharmacies (Fig. 8-5).

Brushing Agents

Various chemical agents have been proposed for the removal and prevention of plaque in humans and animals. Unfortunately, a 100%-effective agent has yet to be

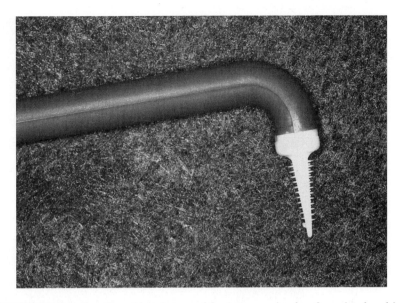

FIGURE 8-5 A fine-tipped brush is used for interproximal or furcation brushing.

developed; therefore brushing is still the preferred method. Plain water or beef or chicken broth can be used initially to help the patient become accustomed to brushing. Sometimes, the addition of garlic powder to the water helps. The mechanical action of brushing or wiping is the important factor in plaque control, not the agent itself.

Home-Care Products

The number of dental home-care products is increasing steadily, and all claim to be effective. Unfortunately, little research exists to prove efficacy. In 1997 the American Veterinary Dental College formed the Veterinary Oral Health Council (VOHC). This organization was established to set testing protocol. If product testing is approved, the product is awarded the VOHC seal of approval.

Enzyme toothpastes

Canine Enzymatic Toothpaste (C.E.T.®) reportedly enhances and activates the natural defense mechanisms of the mouth by providing key catalysts and antiplaque chemicals (Fig. 8-6). In addition to abrasive materials, glucose oxidase and lactoperoxidase are chemicals that combine to produce the hypothiocyanite ion, which is the same ion produced naturally in saliva to help inhibit bacterial growth. C.E.T.® Forte Enzymatic Dentifrice for Cats has a seafood flavor, and C.E.T.® Forte for Dogs has a beef flavor, both of which are designed to appeal to the respective species (Figs. 8-7 and 8-8). Heska™ Theradontic® paste contains sodium monofluorophosphate, glucose oxidase, and lactoperoxidase.

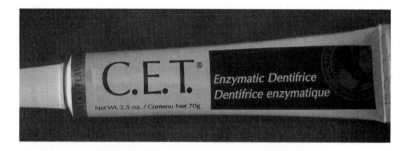

FIGURE 8-6 C.E.T.® Enzymatic Toothpaste.

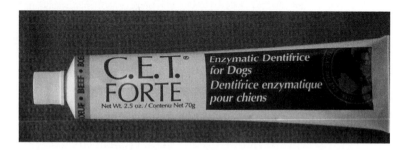

FIGURE 8-7 C.E.T.® Forte for dogs.

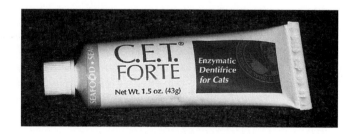

FIGURE 8-8 C.E.T.® Forte for cats.

Antibacterial and anticalculus products

The DentiVet™ (Virbac®) products contain the plaque-controlling agents chlorhexidine gluconate, zinc, and sodium hexametaphosphate (Fig. 8-9). All these chemicals have properties that either combat plaque or inhibit the formation of calculus.

Antibacterial products
Chlorhexidine

An increasing number of products contain chlorhexidine. The advantage of chlorhexidine is its substantivity, or its ability to adhere to oral tissues and release its agents slowly. Heska Theradontic Rinse contains chlorhexidine gluconate. CHX® Guard LA is chlorhexidine gluconate in a malt-flavored gel form that easily coats the oral cavity (Fig. 8-10). The active ingredient in CHX® Guard Oral Rinsing Solution is chlorhexidine gluconate. Novadent™ contains chlorhexidine acetate.

Zinc

Zinc ascorbate (Maxiguard) is effective in the elimination of plaque and the stimulation of healing. The canine formula of Maxiguard contains vitamin C and zinc sulfate. The feline formula contains vitamin C, zinc sulfate, and taurine. Maxiguard is available as a liquid, which is sprayed in the oral cavity, or as a gel, which is applied with a cotton-tipped applicator (Fig. 8-11).

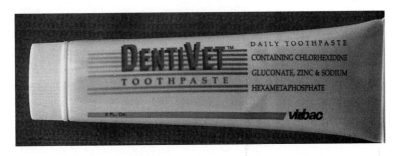

FIGURE 8-9 DentiVet™ toothpaste.

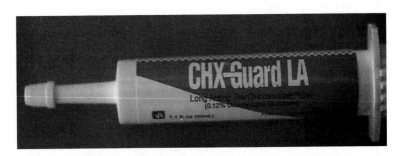

FIGURE 8-10 CHX® Guard LA (long-acting).

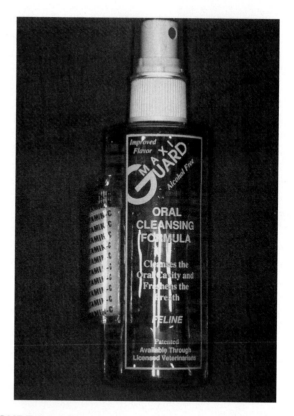

FIGURE 8-11 Maxiguard is available in spray and gel formula.

Fluoride gels

Several types of fluoride are available. Stannous fluoride, the most bactericidal agent, is stable at a pH of 6.5. The 0.4% strength should be used. Fluoride has been shown to aid in plaque prevention when deposited on the surface of the enamel. Although it is unlikely to cause toxicity in this strength, the client should be cautioned to use the product sparingly. Any food in the stomach at the time of ingestion will likely neutralize the fluoride. MFP fluoride is the form of fluoride most commonly found in over-the-counter products. Because of its acid content, this product is not recommended for home care. The product most commonly used is Flurofom® (Virbac), which is a foam. Table 8-1 summarizes the various home-care products available.

Selecting the Appropriate Home-Care Product

The type of dental product recommended depends on the severity of the pathologic condition. For those patients whose oral health is good (e.g., Stage 1 or Stage 2), the priority is to begin the brushing procedure. For these patients, starting out with flavored animal toothpastes, such as VRx® C.E.T.®, Virbac® DentiVet®, or Heska Theradontic™ paste®, establishes the routine. For patients with Stage 3 peri-

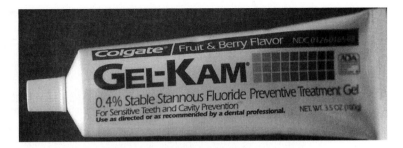

FIGURE 8-12 Gel-Kam stannous fluoride gel.

TABLE 8-1 Tooth-Brushing Agents

Product	Manufacturer	Active ingredients
C.E.T.® Mint, Malt, and Poultry Flavor	Virbac Corporation	Glucose oxidase, lactoperoxidase
C.E.T.® Forte (Canine)	Virbac Corporation	Glucose oxidase, lactoperoxidase
C.E.T.® Forte (Feline)	Virbac Corporation	Glucose oxidase, lactoperoxidase
Heska™ Daily Dental Rinse	Heska	0.12% chlorhexidine gluconate; zinc gluconate
Theradontic™ Rinse®	Heska	Zinc-free chlorhexidine gluconate
Theradontic™ Paste®	Heska	Sodium monofluorophosphate, glucose oxidase, lactoperoxidase
Novadent™ Solution	Fort Dodge	Chlorhexidine acetate
CHX® Guard LA Solution	Virbac Corporation	Chlorhexidine gluconate
CHX® Guard LA Gel	Virbac Corporation	Chlorhexidine gluconate
DentiVet®	Virbac Corporation	Chlorhexidine gluconate, zinc, sodium hexametaphosphate
Maxiguard™ (Canine)	Addison Labs	Vitamin C, zinc sulfate
Maxiguard™ (Feline)	Addison Labs	Vitamin C, zinc sulfate, taurine
Gel-Kam®	Colgate	Stannous fluoride

odontal disease, the introduction of a fluoride product for plaque control becomes more important. The use of flavored animal toothpastes to establish the routine interjected with twice-weekly treatments with stannous fluoride to help inhibit plaque formation is advised. Patients with Stage 4 periodontal disease need more help at home; coating the mouth with chlorhexidine gel and rinsing the mouth with a chlorhexidine solution twice daily for 2 weeks may be beneficial. At the end of the 2-week period a stannous fluoride gel is substituted for the chlorhexidine (Fig. 8-12). All patients may benefit from the use of a zinc ascorbate spray 1 to 4 times daily.

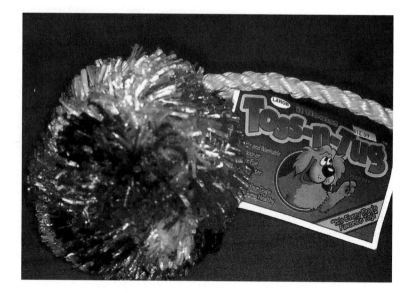

FIGURE 8-13 Toss-n-Tug® chew toy.

OTHER HOME-CARE AIDS

Clients frequently ask how often they should brush their pets' teeth. Because of the way plaque and calculus form, daily brushing is best. Plaque forms 6 to 8 hours after brushing. Bacteria attach to the tooth and aid in the formation of calculus in 3 to 5 days. The client advised to brush the teeth every other day may indeed do so. However, clients are prone to the human tendency of procrastination. Every other day stretches to every 3 days, and at that point calculus may form.

Plaque-Removing Chew Toys

Clients frequently ask veterinary staff to recommend chew toys. Objects such as pig ears and hooves, bones, and other animal parts are simply too hard and will fracture teeth. Toss-n-Tug®, Boodabones, Kong toys, "Pull" or "Pool" toys are all acceptable products (Fig. 8-13). However, the client must be reminded that all toys should be used under proper supervision.

Plaque-Removing Chews

Some plaque-removing chews help retard the formation of plaque by virtue of their formulation. Studies have shown that Dentabone™, C.E.T. Chews™, and Waltham Tartar Chews™ all inhibit the formation of plaque and tartar (Figs. 8-14 and 8-15).

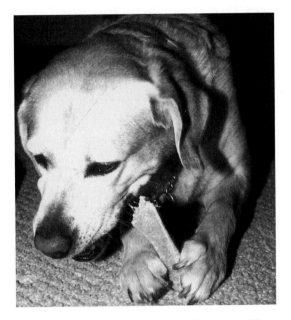

FIGURE 8-14 Dog chewing a Dentabone™.

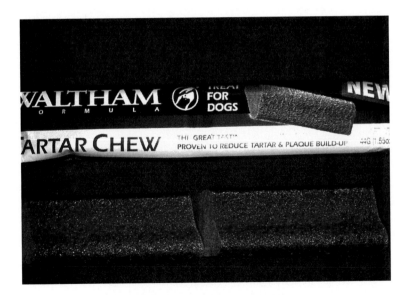

FIGURE 8-15 Waltham Tartar Chews.

Foods That Decrease Plaque Formation

Some foods promote cleansing of the teeth. Dentabone™, T/D™ (Canine and Feline), Milkbone Dog Biscuits™, and Friskies Feline Dental Diet are examples of this type of product. In general, dry food, by virtue of its texture (which increases salivary flow), is better than canned dog food at inhibiting plaque.

Worksheet

STUDENT NAME: _____

1. Client education should begin _____ the procedure is performed.

2. If possible, a "_____" dog (or cat) should be used to demonstrate tooth brushing to the client.

3. A circular motion with emphasis on the _____ stroke is recommended to demonstrate tooth brushing to the client.

4. _____ _____ and _____ _____ are also beneficial in reinforcing the need for brushing and home care.

5. The most important strategy in the prevention of periodontal disease is _____ _____.

6. In 1997 the American Veterinary Dental College formed the _____ _____ _____ _____.

7. The advantage of _____ is its substantivity.

8. The client must be reminded that all toys should be used under _____ _____.

9. _____ brushing is advised.

10. Plaque forms _____ to _____ hours after brushing.

9

Periodontal Therapy

The primary objective of periodontal therapy is the treatment of periodontal disease. The difference between preventive dentistry and dentistry for the treatment of disease is important. As discussed in Chapter 7, a prophylaxis, or prophy, is performed on patients with Stage 1 (early gingivitis) or Stage 2 (advanced gingivitis) as the prevention of periodontal disease. Periodontal therapy, which is nonsurgical, is used in the treatment of patients with Stage 3 (early periodontitis) and Stage 4 (advanced periodontitis) periodontal disease. Root planing, the traditional method of treatment, differs from scaling and the newer form of treatment, periodontal debridement.

SCALING

Scaling is the mechanical removal of plaque, calculus, and stains from the crown and root surfaces. The act of scaling does not necessarily treat periodontal disease. It only removes the surface irritants. The technique for scaling is discussed in Chapter 7, in the section that deals with gross calculus removal.

ROOT PLANING

Root planing is more definitive than scaling. The objective of root planing is the removal of calculus and cementum from the root surface and the creation of a clean, smooth, glasslike root surface. In this treatment, everything, including cementum, is removed from the root surface.

Root Planing: Technique

A routine, systematic approach should be used on each quadrant and each tooth. The blade of the curette is positioned against the root surface. Root planing is performed using a curette with overlapping strokes in horizontal, vertical, and oblique directions (Fig. 9-1). This cross-hatch planing creates an optimally smooth surface and maintains root anatomy.

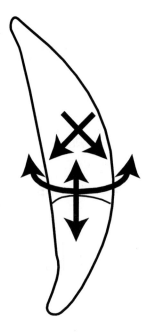

FIGURE 9-1 Cross-hatching strokes performed in root planing to create a smooth surface.

PERIODONTAL DEBRIDEMENT

Periodontal debridement is the treatment of gingival and periodontal inflammation. Its goal is the mechanical removal of surface irritants while maintaining soft tissue and allowing it to return to a healthy, noninflamed state.

Changes in Instrumentation Theory

Theories have changed with regard to root-planing techniques and instruments. Most experts no longer recommend the complete stripping of the dentin surface. This change in theory came about with the increased availability of higher-frequency ultrasonic scalers and thinner tips. Unlike the wider tips used in ultrasonic scaling for gross calculus removal, the newer tips are thinner and can enter the periodontal pocket with less distention of the gingiva and less risk of harm to the tissues, which sometimes occurs with curettes. *[Pockets, periodontal. An area of diseased gingival attachment, characterized by loss of attachment and eventual damage to the tooth's supporting bone.]* Proper use of the new ultrasonic instruments is much easier. In addition, newer antimicrobials and antibiotics are available for use in treatment.

Cementum Removal

Cementum is the substance that attaches the periodontal ligament to the tooth. In the past, experts believed that calculus and toxins from bacteria were embedded in the cementum; therefore removal of the cementum was necessary. Newer research has shown that bacterial plaque is loosely bound and molecular growth factors are

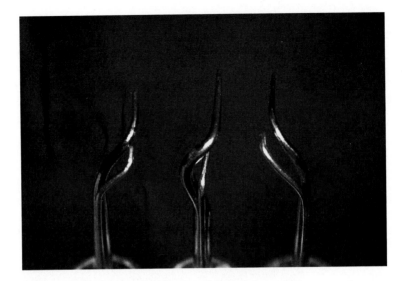

FIGURE 9-2 Ultrasonic tips suitable for subgingival use. Two of these instruments have hooks, allowing them to advance around crowns and into furcations.

contained within the cementum, aiding in the reattachment of the periodontal ligament to the root surface. Now, only the removal of plaque and calculus is mandatory.

Benefits of Ultrasonic Periodontal Therapy

When properly used, ultrasonic scalers remove the least amount of cementum, as compared with sonic scalers or hand instruments. In addition, the ultrasonic scalers provide water lavage that allows better visualization of the tissues and flushes or removes debris from the pocket. Because they irrigate the tissues, ultrasonic scalers also improve cleanliness and wound healing.

Ultrasonic scalers are able to clean the root surface more efficiently than hand instruments. The result is less time on treatment and less time when the patient is under anesthesia. Moreover, the sonic waves produced have a cavitation effect, disrupting the bacterial cell wall.

Ultrasonic periodontal therapy has several advantages over traditional ultrasonic therapy, in which a curette is used. First, because the ultrasonic tip creates less distention of the gingival tissues than a curette, less trauma occurs and healing is faster. No sharpening of the instrument is required. Because there are no cutting edges, the risk of gingival laceration is reduced, making ultrasonic periodontal therapy safer.

Ultrasonic Tips

Several companies (e.g., Dentsply, Parkell, Hu-Friedy Co.) manufacture various types of ultrasonic tips, including the metal-stack–type ultrasonic tip. Generally, the use of shorter tips for shallow pockets and longer tips for deeper pockets is recommended. Some tips have corkscrew-type angles. These are designed to advance around crowns and into furcations (Fig. 9-2).

LOCAL ANTIBIOTIC THERAPY

Antibiotic therapy can be used with periodontal debridement techniques. One product is HESKA™ PERIO*ceutic*® gel, which delivers doxycycline directly to the periodontal pockets. The medication provides local delivery of an antibiotic to afford local control of the microorganisms responsible for periodontal disease. According to the manufacturer, the gel reduces periodontal pocket depth, increases attachment levels, and reduces gingival inflammation. The two-syringe system necessitates mixing before use. Syringe A contains the polymer delivery system, and Syringe B contains the active ingredient (doxycycline) (Fig. 9-3).

The A and B syringes should be connected to each other. The material is transferred back and forth 100 times, then inserted into a pocket with the provided cannula (Fig. 9-4). The gel hardens when exposed to water (Fig. 9-5). The hardened material is packed into the pocket with a plastic working instrument (Figs. 9-6 and 9-7).

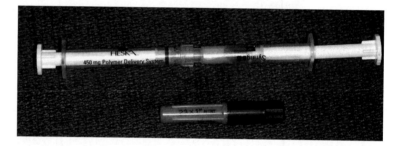

FIGURE 9-3 HESKA™ PERIO*ceutic*® syringes A and B attached with periodontal needle.

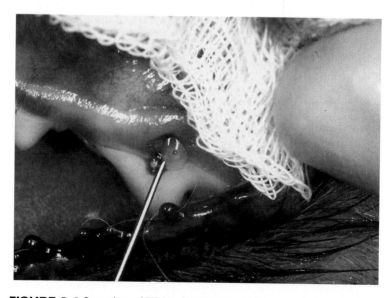

FIGURE 9-4 Insertion of HESKA™ PERIO*ceutic*® into periodontal pocket.

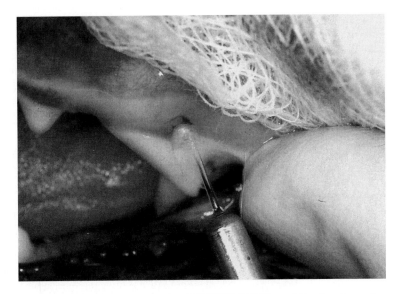

FIGURE 9-5 Water irrigating HESKA™ PERIO*ceutic*® to harden gel.

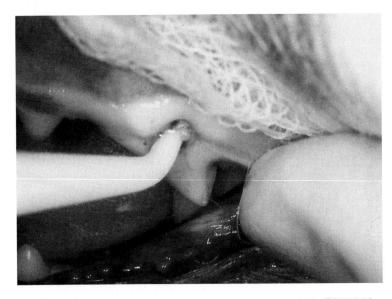

FIGURE 9-6 Plastic working instrument being used to pack HESKA™ PERIO*ceutic*® into pocket.

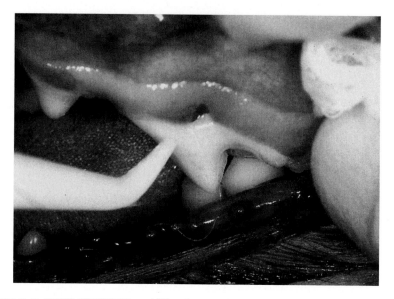

FIGURE 9-7 HESKA™ PERIO*ceutic*® has been packed into this periodontal pocket at the furcation.

HESKA™ PERIO*ceutic*® gel is indicated for the treatment and control of periodontal disease in dogs. Depths greater than or equal to 4 mm in the periodontal pockets are evidence of disease that may respond to treatment with HESKA™ PERIO*ceutic*® gel. As a medical treatment, this procedure should be performed by the veterinarian.

CONCLUSION

Good follow-up procedures are necessary for the treatment of patients with periodontal disease. The treatment plan is revised as necessary.

Worksheet

STUDENT NAME: _____

1. The primary objective of periodontal therapy is to

   _____ _____ _____.

2. Periodontal therapy is performed on patients with Stage

   _____ or Stage _____ periodontal

   disease.

3. _____ is the mechanical removal of plaque,

   calculus, and stains from the crown and root surfaces.

4. The objective of _____ _____ is to

   create a clean, smooth, glasslike root surface.

5. Root planing is performed using a curette with overlapping

   strokes in _____, _____, and

   _____ directions.

6. _____ _____ is the treatment of gingival

   and periodontal inflammation.

7. Newer research has shown that it is no longer necessary to

   remove _____.

8. The sonic waves produced by ultrasonic scalers have a

   cavitation effect, _____ the bacterial cell wall.

9. HESKA™ PERIO*ceutic*® gel delivers _____ directly to

   the periodontal pocket.

10. HESKA™ PERIO*ceutic*® gel should be mixed _____

    times before use.

10

Exodontics (Extractions)

Although the object in veterinary dentistry is to save teeth, extraction often becomes necessary. Exodontics is the branch of dentistry that involves the extraction of teeth.

INDICATIONS FOR EXODONTICS

Exodontics is indicated when the tooth cannot be salvaged or the client is unable or unwilling to perform home care. The client should be consulted for authorization before any teeth are extracted. In addition to becoming upset with the extra fees, clients may respond emotionally to their pets' loss of teeth. Alternative types of treatment should always be discussed. Staff members must always remember that extraction is final.

THE TECHNICIAN AND EXTRACTIONS

With regard to extraction, laws vary from state to state. In all states, if extraction by someone other than a veterinarian is permitted, the extraction must be performed under a veterinarian's supervision. Some state regulations are contradictory. For example, in some states, registered veterinary technicians are permitted to perform extractions. However, the law forbids registered veterinary technicians from performing surgery. Many extractions are surgical (e.g., when teeth are split, flaps performed). This presents a conflict for the technician. The safe position, if allowed by state law and the veterinarian, is for the technician to perform only nonsurgical extractions, such as removal of extremely mobile teeth.

The American Veterinary Dental College (AVDC), which represents board-certified veterinary dental specialists throughout the world, has evaluated the duties of the veterinarian, registered veterinary technician, and nonlicensed individuals in practice. As a result, the AVDC developed a position statement stipulating that only veterinarians should provide extraction services (Box 10-1).

BOX 10-1

American Veterinary Dental College (AVDC) Position Statement Regarding Veterinary Dental Healthcare Providers (Adopted April 5, 1998)

The AVDC has developed this position as a means to safeguard the veterinary dental patient and to ensure the qualifications of persons performing veterinary dental procedures.

Primary responsibility for veterinary dental care

The AVDC defines veterinary dentistry as the art and practice of oral health care in animals other than man. It is a discipline of veterinary medicine and surgery. The diagnosis, treatment, and management of veterinary oral health care is to be provided and supervised by licensed veterinarians or by veterinarians working within a university or industry.

Who may provide veterinarian-supervised dental care

The AVDC accepts that the following health-care workers may assist the responsible veterinarian in dental procedures or actually perform dental prophylactic services while under direct, in-the-room supervision by a veterinarian if permitted by local law: licensed, certified, or registered veterinary technician; a veterinary assistant with advanced dental training; dentist; and registered dental hygienist.

Operative dentistry and oral surgery

The AVDC considers operative dentistry to be any dental procedure that invades the hard or soft oral tissue including, but not limited to, a procedure that alters the structure of one or more teeth or repairs damaged and diseased teeth. A veterinarian should perform operative dentistry and oral surgery.

Extraction of teeth

The AVDC considers the extraction of teeth to be included in the practice of veterinary dentistry. Decision-making is the responsibility of the veterinarian, with the consent of the pet owner, when electing to extract teeth. Only veterinarians shall determine which teeth are to be extracted and perform extraction procedures.

BOX 10-1

American Veterinary Dental College (AVDC) Position Statement Regarding Veterinary Dental Healthcare Providers (Adopted April 5, 1998)—cont'd

Dental tasks performed by veterinary technicians

The AVDC considers it appropriate for a veterinarian to delegate maintenance dental care and certain dental tasks to a veterinary technician. Tasks appropriately performed by a technician include dental prophylaxis and certain procedures that do not result in altering the shape, structure, or positional location of teeth in the dental arch. The veterinarian may direct a technician to perform these tasks provided that the veterinarian is physically present and supervising the treatment and provided that the technician has received appropriate training.

The AVDC supports the advanced training of veterinary technicians to perform additional ancillary dental services: taking impressions, making models, charting veterinary dental pathology, taking and developing dental radiographs, performing nonsurgical subgingival root scaling and debridement, providing that they do not alter the structure of the tooth.

Tasks that may be performed by veterinary assistants (not registered, certified, or licensed)

The AVDC supports the appropriate training of veterinary assistants to perform the following dental services: supragingival scaling and polishing, taking and developing dental radiographs, making impressions, and making models.

Tasks that may be performed by dentists, registered dental hygienists, and other dental health-care providers

The AVDC recognizes that dentists, registered dental hygienists, and other dental health-care providers in good standing may perform those procedures for which they have been qualified under the direct supervision of the veterinarian. The supervising veterinarian will be responsible for the welfare of the patient and any treatment performed on the patient.

The AVDC understands that individual states have regulations that govern the practice of veterinary medicine. This position statement is intended to be a model for veterinary dental practice and does not replace existing law.

INSTRUMENTS FOR EXODONTICS

A variety of instruments are used for extractions (Box 10-2). Dental elevators are used to engage teeth and raise them from the root socket. Extraction forceps grasp the tooth and remove it from the socket (Fig. 10-1).

Elevators and Root Tip Picks

Because teeth vary in size, a variety of sizes of dental elevators is necessary (Fig. 10-2). To add to the confusion, different manufacturers use different names and number-

---

BOX 10-2
Instruments for Exodontics

Surgical extraction: scalpel handle with blade (11 blade, 15c)
Periosteal elevator: Molt No. 2 (small patient) or Molt No. 4 (large patient)
Burs: tapered crosscut bur, No. 701L for sectioning multiroot tooth
Dental elevators: 301SS, 301S, 301, 34
Root tip picks: Miltex 78, HB 10/11, Heidbrink
Irrigation solution: Sterile saline, dilute chlorhexidine solution
Periodontal scissors to release flap
Needle holder
Thumb forceps
Resorbable suture with swaged needle
Suture scissors
Bone implant material: Consil®
Dental radiographic material

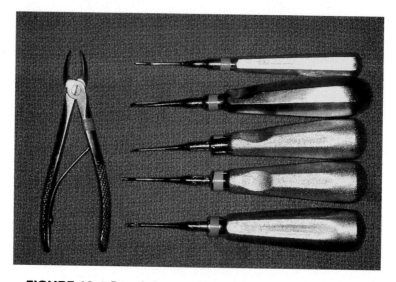

FIGURE 10-1 Dental elevators *(right)* and extraction forceps *(left)*.

ing systems to identify their instruments. The 301, 301s, and 301ss types are fine elevators. The 301s is especially useful in extracting feline teeth. The 301ss elevators are even smaller. All the elevators in the 301 series have been modified by notching the back side of the instrument, creating a fork to assist in preventing the instrument from sliding off alveolar crests (Fig. 10-3). The 301ss are effective in elevating small teeth in cats. The 301s are effective in elevating primary canine teeth in dogs

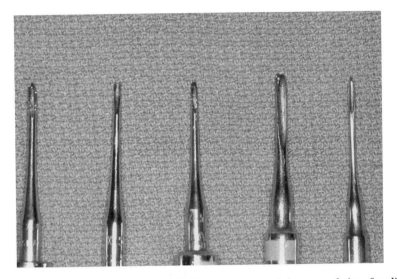

FIGURE 10-2 Dental elevators are available in a variety of shapes and sizes for different sized and shaped teeth.

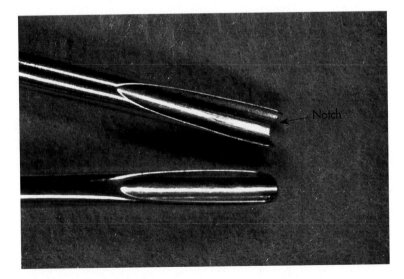

FIGURE 10-3 A notch has been created in the upper instrument that helps to prevent it from slipping off the alveolar crest.

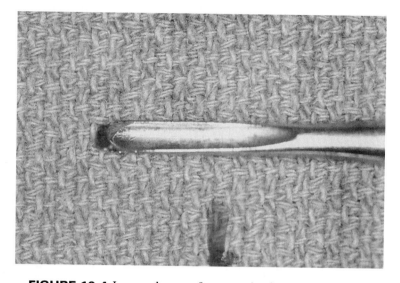

FIGURE 10-4 Larger elevators for extracting larger canine teeth.

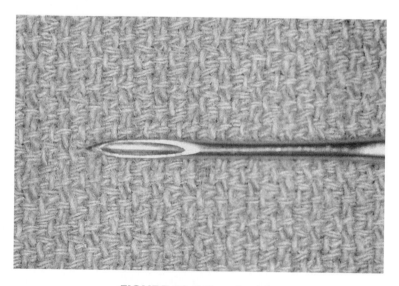

FIGURE 10-5 Root tip pick.

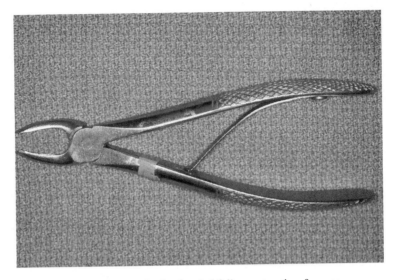

FIGURE 10-6 Spring-loaded feline extraction forceps.

and premolars in cats. The 301 is effective in elevating canine teeth in cats and incisors and premolars in dogs. Medium-sized elevators are used for elevating larger premolar roots and moderate-sized canine teeth in dogs. Large elevators are used in extracting larger canine teeth in dogs (Fig.10-4).

The Heidbrink root tip pick, HB10/11, and Miltex 78 are useful in elevating and extracting retained root tips. They also can be used to cut the gingival attachment from the tooth before elevation with dental elevators (Fig. 10-5).

Extraction Forceps

Smaller extraction forceps are designed for dog and cat teeth. They are much easier to use than the type used on humans. Use of spring-loaded forceps is recommended (Fig. 10-6).

Magnification and Lighting

One frustrating aspect of root extraction is limited access and visibility. This problem may be decreased by the use of magnification ($\times3$) and head lamps.

STERILIZATION OF EQUIPMENT

Because extraction is a surgical procedure and the instrument enters tissue, sterile instruments should always be used (Fig. 10-7). Although most often the tissue around the tooth is already infected, use of a nonsterile instrument could introduce a different species of bacteria to the infection. Chemical disinfectants may be effective, but they take time to work and necessitate complete cleaning of the instrument

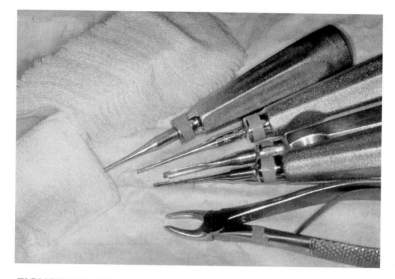

FIGURE 10-7 Extraction instruments should be sterilized before use.

before use. Moreover, chemical sterilization can dull sharp instruments and weaken some metals. Gas sterilization techniques do not cause as much damage to the instruments. However, the gases must be properly used to prevent heath hazards. Autoclaving techniques use a combination of pressure and steam heat to sterilize instruments.

Sterilization Monitoring

Sterilization must be monitored, either with chemical strips that turn colors when the proper sterile conditions have been achieved or with biologic monitors in which bacterial growth is observed after sterilization.

EXODONTIC PRINCIPLES

The tooth may be removed from the socket in two ways. The force technique breaks bone (and tooth root) and causes more trauma than necessary; its use is therefore discouraged. The best approach is to stretch and tear the periodontal ligament fibers. The use of elevators to fracture bone by excessive force is not recommended. Often, both bone and root are fractured, which causes excessive trauma. A rotational motion (rather than a "seesaw" motion) should be used. The tooth should be eased out of the socket rather than forced. The key to this approach is patience.

Root Removal

All of the root should be removed, except in the rare instance when more root retrieval would cause more damage. With any extraction procedure, dental radiographs help ensure that all the root tissue has been removed.

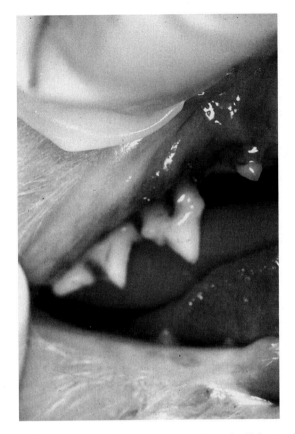

FIGURE 10-8 The gingiva has been elevated off the tooth.

Exodontic Technique

A step-by-step approach in exodontic technique is important. Practitioners must always remember that the object is to remove the tooth with as little trauma as possible. Use of each of these techniques may not be necessary for every extraction, nor is the order of steps necessarily followed each time. Combinations of vertical and horizontal extraction may be used.

Single-root extraction

Single-rooted teeth in the dog are the incisors, canines, first premolars, and mandibular third molar; in the cat, they are the incisors, canines, and maxillary second premolar. The cat's maxillary first molar may be treated as a single-rooted tooth even though it has more than one root. The first step in tooth extraction is to sever the gingival attachment (Fig. 10-8). A root tip pick or dental elevator is most commonly used. The practitioner should work all the way around the tooth and remember to be patient.

Occasionally, use of a round or pear-shaped bur on a high-speed handpiece may be helpful in separating the ligament. Plenty of water should be used to keep the tissues cool; otherwise, bone necrosis could result from excessive heating of the bone.

Vertical rotation

In vertical rotation the elevator is used parallel to the root (Fig. 10-9). Once the free gingiva *[Free gingiva. Portion of the gingiva not directly attached to the tooth that forms the gingival wall of the sulcus.]* has been severed, the practitioner should begin to work an elevator, whose curve approximates the tooth, into the space between the tooth and the alveolus. Placing a slow, gentle, steady pressure on the tooth rather than quick, rocking motions is helpful. The slow, steady pressure (holding the pressure on each side 5 to 15 seconds may be necessary) will break down the periodontal ligament so that the tooth exfoliates easily.

Horizontal rotation

In horizontal rotation the elevator is placed perpendicular to the crown and tooth root. Pressure is applied to the coronal aspect of the tooth to be extracted. Care should be taken not to luxate the tooth that is acting as a fulcrum (Fig. 10-10). When the periodontal ligament breaks down, the tooth is held with extraction forceps for easy removal (Fig. 10-11). To increase the speed of healing, the socket and associated gingiva should be cleaned by curettage and irrigation.

Bone augmentation

A synthetic material (Consil®, Nutramax Laboratories) is available to fill in the socket after the tooth is extracted.

Suturing

Finally, the gingiva is sutured using 3-0 or 4-0 synthetic suture material. Maxon™, Vicryl™, or Dexon™ is recommended because these types dissolve or become untied and fall out in several weeks.

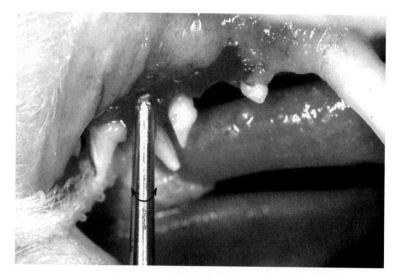

FIGURE 10-9 Vertical rotational movement of the instrument.

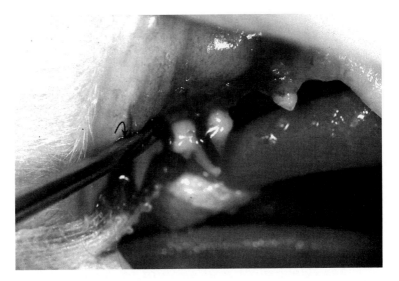

FIGURE 10-10 Without luxating adjoining teeth, horizontal luxation is used to avulse the tooth to be extracted coronally.

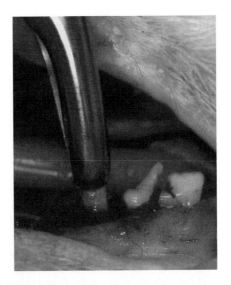

FIGURE 10-11 After the periodontal ligament is broken down, extraction forceps are used to remove the tooth from the socket.

Multirooted teeth

Splitting multirooted teeth before extracting them is almost always the easiest method. After the teeth are split, each section should be removed as if it were a single-rooted tooth.

Premolar extraction

All premolars except the first (one root) and the maxillary fourth should be split by using a high-speed bur to cut between the furcation and the tip of the crown (Fig. 10-12).

Maxillary fourth premolar

The maxillary fourth premolar should be separated between the furcations and the crown of each of the three roots. The first cut is made between the cusps over the mesial-buccal and distal roots (Fig. 10-13). The second cut is made to separate the mesial-buccal and palatal roots (Fig. 10-14).

Maxillary first and second molars

In dogs a T-shaped cut can be made on the maxillary first and second molars. This T should first split off the mesial and distal roots from the palatine root, and then separate the mesial and distal roots (Fig. 10-15). Once the crown has been split, each individual root is treated as a separate tooth and extracted. The only difference with this technique is that adjoining roots may be used as fulcrums for the extraction before and after the root has been elevated.

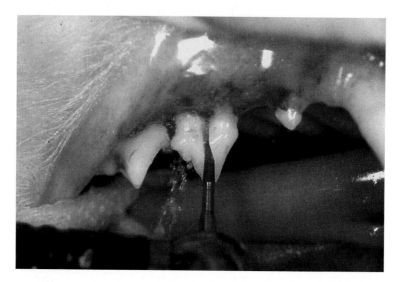

FIGURE 10-12 A high-speed bur is used to cut the crown, splitting the tooth into two single-root sections.

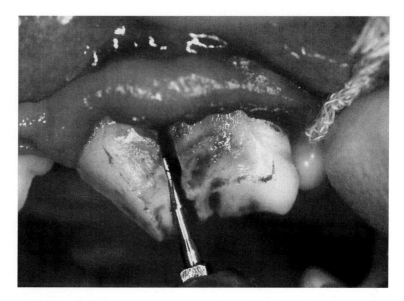

FIGURE 10-13 The first incision is made with a high-speed handpiece to separate the tooth's mesial-buccal and distal roots.

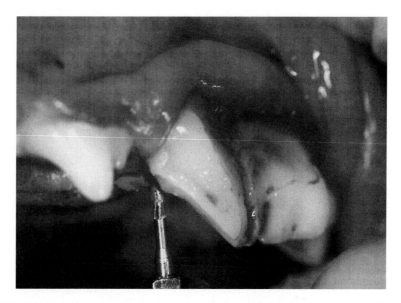

FIGURE 10-14 The second incision is made between the mesial-buccal and palatal roots.

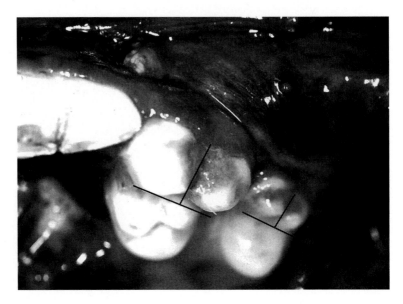

FIGURE 10-15 In dogs a T-shaped cut can be made on the first and second molars to split the tooth into three sections.

EXTRACTION COMPLICATIONS

Complications may occur while extracting teeth. Occasionally, stubborn roots or root tips remain. The roots may be difficult to extract. The preferred treatment in this situation is to create a flap and elevate the tooth buccally.

Flap Surgery

Releasing incisions are made on the mesial-buccal and distal buccal line angles of adjacent teeth. These releasing incisions are joined by an intrasulcular incision that follows the gingival margin. The gingiva is stripped from the bone with a periosteal elevator. The buccal plate of bone over the tooth is removed with a high-speed handpiece and irrigation. The root is removed, and the flap is closed.

Pulverization

An alternative to flap surgery is to use a high-speed handpiece with a pear-shaped, round, or crosscut fissure bur to pulverize the remaining root. A word of caution however: The practitioner must be sure to use plenty of water spray to keep the tissues cool. Burned bone (apparent by its odor) can lead to the future problems of necrosis and slow healing at the extraction site. In most cases, leaving the root intact is preferable to pulverizing it.

CONCLUSION

Most exodontic procedures are surgical extractions. If permitted by law and practice policy, the technician should receive advanced, hands-on training of exodontic technique. Great harm can be done to patients when inexperienced or untrained staff members perform these procedures.

Worksheet

STUDENT NAME: _____

1. Exodontics may be indicated if the tooth is judged nonsalvageable or if the client is unable or unwilling to perform _____.

2. The client should be consulted for _____ before any teeth are extracted.

3. With regard to extraction, _____ vary from state to state.

4. The law of some states permits _____ of teeth by registered veterinary technicians.

5. The law of some states forbids registered veterinary technicians from performing _____.

6. _____ _____ are instruments that are used to engage teeth and raise them from the root socket.

7. _____ are used to grasp the tooth and remove it from the socket.

8. The _____, _____, and _____ are fine elevators and are good for extracting very small teeth.

9. The _____ root tip pick and HB10/11 root tip picks are useful in extracting retained root tips.

10. Use of _____ _____ forceps is recommended.

11. Because extraction is a surgical procedure and the instrument often enters tissue, _____ _____ should be used.

12. The _____ technique breaks bone (and tooth root) and causes more trauma than necessary.

13. The use of elevators to fracture bone by excessive force is _____.

14. A _____ motion rather than a "seesaw" motion should be used.

15. _____-rooted teeth are the incisors, the canines, the first premolars, and mandibular third molar in the dog, and the incisors, canines, and maxillary second premolar in the cat.

16. In _____ rotation the elevator parallel to the root is used.

17. Splitting _____ teeth before extracting them is almost always the easiest method.

18. A _____ -shaped cut can be made on the maxillary first molar.

19. _____ _____ may be helpful in making sure that all the root tissue has been removed.

20. Occasionally, stubborn roots or root tips remain. The preferred treatment in this situation is to create a _____ and elevate the tooth buccally.

11

Dental Radiology

Dental radiography may be used in all veterinary offices. Although dental radiography is surrounded by a great deal of mystique, it is not extremely difficult to master, given time and practice.

INDICATIONS FOR DENTAL RADIOGRAPHY

Dental radiographs may be used to document and study the progress of therapeutic programs in the treatment of all types of dental and oral diseases. When neoplasia or metabolic disease is suspected, radiographs may be used to evaluate the involvement of teeth and bone; in cases of oral trauma, radiographs are helpful in the evaluation of the mandible and maxilla.

Unerupted or Impacted Teeth

In young patients, radiographs help the practitioner determine whether unerupted or impacted teeth are present (Fig. 11-1). *[Impacted tooth. An unerupted or partially erupted tooth that is prevented from erupting further by any structure.]* Dental radiographs are taken in all patients to evaluate the status of root and tooth when the tooth is missing or partly erupted. The practitioner may discover that the patient is edentulous or has a dilacerated or an imbedded tooth. *[Edentulous. The absence of teeth.]* *[Dilaceration. An abnormally shaped root resulting from trauma during tooth development.]* *[Embedded. A tooth that is usually covered in bone, has not erupted into the oral cavity, and is not likely to erupt.]*

Periodontal Disease

During prophylactic or therapeutic teeth cleaning, radiographs can be used to determine the extent of periodontal disease. Dental radiographs allow the practitioner to evaluate bone loss and select an appropriate method of treatment. In patients with oral stomas (fistulas), radiographs can also be used as a diagnostic tool.

223

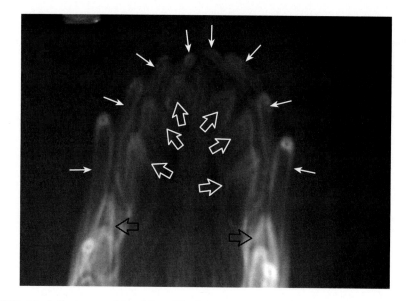

FIGURE 11-1 Both sets of dentition. The large arrows indicate adult teeth, and the small arrows indicate primary (deciduous) teeth.

Endodontics

Radiographs allow the practitioner to evaluate the effectiveness of endodontic therapy and to study radicular health and size before, during, and after endodontic therapy. In patients with missing teeth, radiographs are used to ascertain the status of possibly impacted roots or teeth.

Exodontics

Dental radiographs are indicated before extractions for diagnosis and evaluation of possible complications. Dental radiographs are obtained during the procedure to determine the presence of retained roots and other complications. Radiographs are indicated after extraction to ensure completeness of the procedure.

CONTRAINDICATION FOR DENTAL RADIOLOGY

Dental radiology is contraindicated in critical patients that may have difficulty undergoing anesthesia, which is necessary to allow proper patient positioning. Dental radiology may be used in diagnosis, documentation of progress, and referral consultation.

DENTAL RADIOGRAPHIC EQUIPMENT AND MATERIALS

Veterinary Medical Machines

Dental radiographs can be taken using veterinary medical radiographic units. However, these require considerable effort in positioning the patient. With the stationary radiographic unit, the patient must be moved several times to reorient the head.

Dental Machines

The advantage of the dental radiographic unit is its fairly flexible radiographic head and jointed extension arm. The unit can be angled, which minimizes the need for patient repositioning. Human nature being as it is, practitioners tend to take more radiographs when the unit is easy to use. The greater the number of radiographs, the greater the amount of diagnostic information.

The kV(p) in most dental radiographic units is fixed and usually does not need to be adjusted. Likewise, the milliamperage (mA) for most units is fixed. Time, however, is a variable that may require adjustment according to the thickness of the area to be studied. Some units measure time in portions of a second. Some set time in impulses (one impulse equals one sixtieth of a second; thirty impulses would equal 0.5 seconds).

Intraoral Film

Intraoral radiographic film is inexpensive, small, and flexible (Fig. 11-2). It fits neatly into the oral cavity, conforming to the area where it is placed. Intraoral film is non-screen film, which provides greater detail than the screen films used in most veterinary situations. Intraoral film can be processed in 1 to 2 minutes in rapid developer and fixer solutions, with minimal loss of detail. This film allows the isolation of small areas of interest.

Description

Most intraoral film comprises a series of layers. A plastic coating covers the external portion. Between the plastic coating and the radiographic film is a layer of paper. The next layer is the radiographic film, sandwiched by another layer of paper. Finally, a layer of lead is followed by another layer of paper that can be peeled from the plastic coating. Some manufacturers have combined the lead and paper layers (Fig. 11-3).

Dental radiographic film sizes

Dental radiographic film is available in a number of sizes. DF-58, which is Size 2 film, is the most common film used in human dentistry. It is also called *periapical film*. In veterinary dentistry this type of film is suitable for small patients. DF-50, or Size 4 film, is also called *occlusal film* and is appropriate for larger patients. For cats, Size 0 may be useful for radiographic evaluation of the mandible.

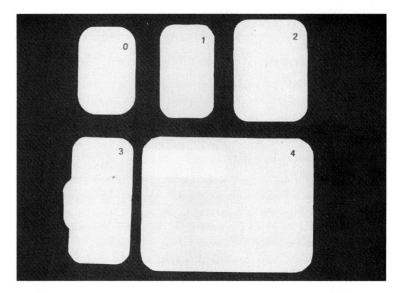

FIGURE 11-2 Several types of intraoral films are available. The author has found the combination of Size 2 (DF-58) and Size 4 (DF-54) to be the most useful.

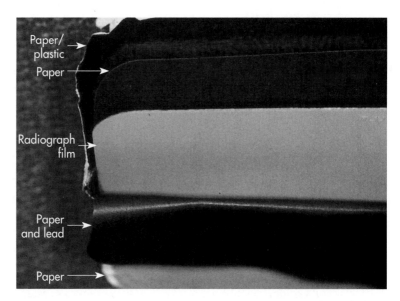

FIGURE 11-3 The intraoral film packet consists of a layer of paper or plastic, paper (next to the film), the radiographic film, another layer of paper, lead (or lead-lined paper), and paper.

Protective Measures

Personnel should protect themselves by wearing lead safety aprons and using screens. They should also maintain a safe distance from the beam of radiation emitted by the radiographic unit. A variety of devices may be used to hold the film in place. Placing the film in holders, resting the film against the endotracheal tube, and securing the film with gauze sponges are a few common methods.

Radiographic Technique

In general, the following tips are helpful to obtain the best technique in setting up for exposure. The distance from the patient should be kept as short as possible. On most radiographic units, the lower mA (e.g., 50 mA) settings use the smaller focal spots. The smaller the focal spot, the sharper the image. The beam of the x-ray unit should be collimated to include only the area of the subject needed.

The following technique is used: First, the radiographic unit control panel is set for the appropriate mA, kV(p), and time. Optimal image is created with a proper balance between kV(p) and mAs. This image will provide a full range of tones from white to black. The practitioner should determine the proper balance. When kVp is low, the result is low density and high contrast. When the kVp is high, the result is very high density with very little contrast. The patient is positioned appropriately for the radiograph to be taken. The intraoral film is placed in the proper position. As an aid in positioning the film, a mouth gag, film wedge, or other object can be placed behind the film. The head of the x-ray machine is placed 8 to 12 inches or as close as possible from the structure being evaluated and positioned for the study. The film is exposed and then developed.

Placing film

The radiographic film should be placed in the mouth so that the plastic side is facing toward the subject and head (position-indicating device) of the radiographic unit. Most radiographic film is printed with a message such as "opposite side toward radiographic unit." A maximal amount of root and supporting bone should be included in the film. Placing the radiographic film in such a way that most of the film is not over tooth and bone is ineffective.

Parallel technique

The parallel technique for oral radiographs is indicated to evaluate the posterior mandibular teeth and nasal cavity. The x-ray film packet is placed parallel to the structure to be radiographed. In the posterior mandible (for mandibular premolar and molar teeth), the x-ray film packet is inserted between the tongue and mandible (Fig. 11-4).

In many areas of the mouth the parallel technique cannot be used. Other structures in the mouth are superimposed on the x-ray film on exposure or prevent the film from being placed parallel to the subject. Examples are the anterior and posterior maxilla, where the hard and soft palates are in the way, and the anterior mandible, where the mandible prevents placing the film parallel to the teeth.

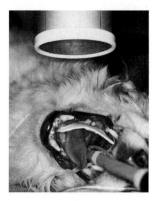

FIGURE 11-4 The parallel technique is used to take radiographs of the mandible.

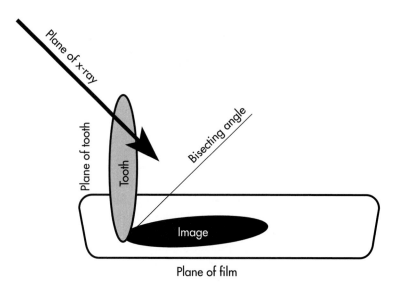

FIGURE 11-5 The plane of the tooth is at a 90-degree angle to the film. The bisecting angle is therefore 45 degrees. The radiographic cone is aimed at this imaginary line. As a result, the image is recorded with slight magnification.

Bisecting angle technique

In the instances described in the previous paragraph, the bisecting angle should be used. The bisecting angle is obtained by visualizing an imaginary line that bisects the angle formed by the x-ray film and the structure being radiographed (Fig. 11-5). If the x-ray beam is aimed at the tooth, the image on the finished film will be distorted by elongation (Fig. 11-6). If the x-ray beam is aimed at the film, the image will also be distorted, this time by foreshortening (Fig. 11-7). To obtain a proper radiograph, the x-ray machine head is positioned so that the beam of the x-ray will be

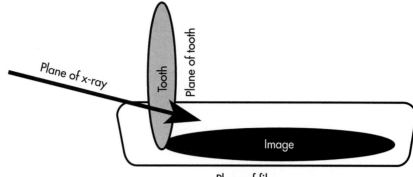

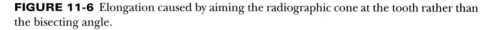

FIGURE 11-6 Elongation caused by aiming the radiographic cone at the tooth rather than the bisecting angle.

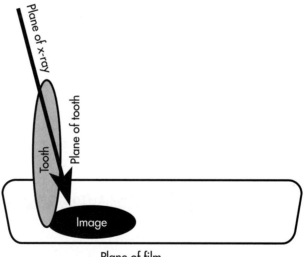

FIGURE 11-7 Foreshortening caused by aiming the radiographic cone toward the film.

perpendicular to the imaginary line. When first learning this technique, some technicians find it helpful to use props, such as sticks (cotton-tipped applicators), to help visualize the bisecting angle.

Spending a lot of time with a protractor to measure all the angles and find the perfect bisecting angle is a waste of effort. Instead, it is easier to follow some simple rules.

Maxillary posterior

For the maxillary posterior teeth (premolars and molars), the film is simply placed across the maxilla parallel to the hard palate. The film is placed so that it does not favor the left or right side; rather, it has an equal margin on both sides of the maxilla. The long end of the film is parallel with the muzzle. Angling the film as close to the hard palate as possible is not important. The patient and radiograph machine head are positioned so that the machine head is 45 degrees off the vertical and horizontal planes of the patient's muzzle (Fig. 11-8).

Maxillary anterior
To radiograph the maxillary anterior teeth, the film is placed in the mouth parallel to the hard palate. The patient and radiograph machine head are positioned so that the machine head is 45 degrees off the vertical and horizontal planes of the patient's muzzle (Fig. 11-9).

Mandibular anterior
To radiograph the mandibular anterior teeth, the film is placed in the mouth parallel to the mandible. The patient is placed in dorsal recumbency, and the radiograph machine head is positioned so that it is 20 degrees off the vertical plane of the anterior mandible or 70 degrees off the horizontal plane of the anterior mandible (Fig. 11-10).

Complete study
The complete radiographic study can be obtained in as little as six views: right and left posterior maxilla, right and left posterior mandible, anterior maxilla, and anterior mandible. Larger patients require additional films to cover all the teeth.

Canine teeth
The canine teeth are best evaluated by placing the machine head 45 degrees from the front of the patient and 45 degrees from the side of the patient (Fig. 11-11).

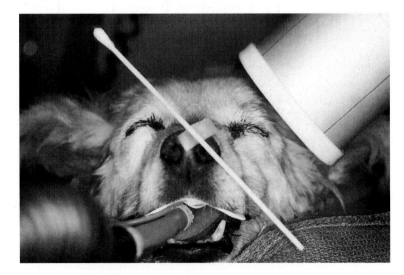

FIGURE 11-8 Maxillary posterior bisecting angle.

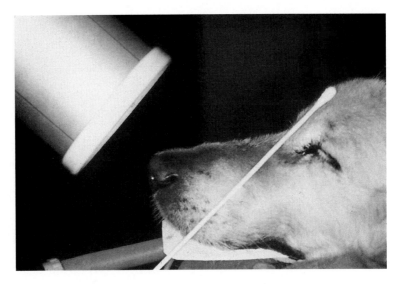

FIGURE 11-9 Maxillary anterior bisecting angle.

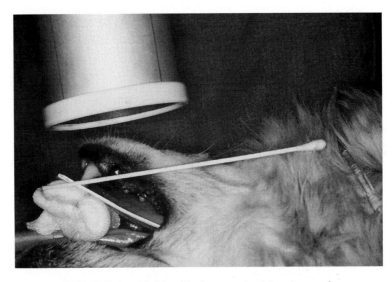

FIGURE 11-10 Mandibular anterior bisecting angle.

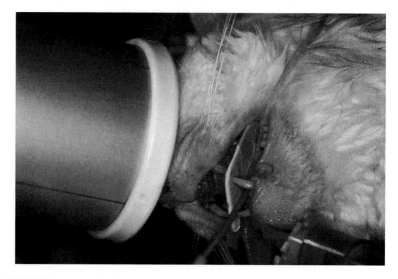

FIGURE 11-11 Radiographic evaluation of the left maxillary canine tooth.

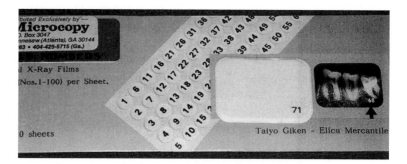

FIGURE 11-12 Numbers can be placed on radiographs before exposure to identify them later.

Marking radiographs

The small size of dental x-ray film can make keeping track of dental radiographs difficult. Once developed and dry, they can be inadvertently shuffled and lost. Micro-copy® makes small radiopaque adhesive numbers for placement on the film packet before exposure. Alternatively, after exposure the film may be written on with radiographic marking pens (Fig. 11-12). The developed films can also be fixed in cardboard or plastic film mounts on which the film, patient, and owner information is written. The dimple on the film should be on the right side of the mouth or upper on the right mandible and lower on the left mandible. In this way the dimple (or number placed next to the dimple) will be "in the air" on the right side and "in the bone" on the left.

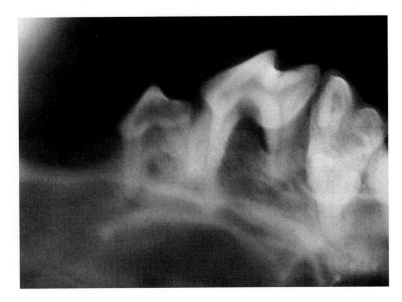

FIGURE 11-13 Blurring caused by movement of the patient or x-ray cone during exposure of the film.

COMPLICATIONS IN DENTAL RADIOLOGY

Complications in dental radiology occur because of improper exposure, positioning, and developing.

Blurred or Double Images

Movement of either the patient or the x-ray machine head causes blurred or double images. If the movement continues throughout the exposure, the image will be blurred. When the film is in one position for part of the exposure and then moved to a second position for the remainder of the exposure, a double image results. Tongue movement in lightly sedated patients may also cause the film to move (Fig. 11-13).

Elongation of Image

If the image appears elongated, the radiographic cone head was probably aimed too directly at the subject as opposed to bisecting the angle between the subject and film. Another possibility is that the film was placed incorrectly (Fig. 11-14).

Foreshortening of Image

If the image appears foreshortened, the radiographic cone head may have been aimed too directly at the radiographic film as opposed to the bisecting angle. Another cause is improper positioning of the film (Fig. 11-15).

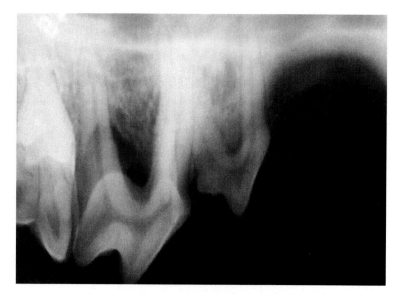

FIGURE 11-14 Elongation.

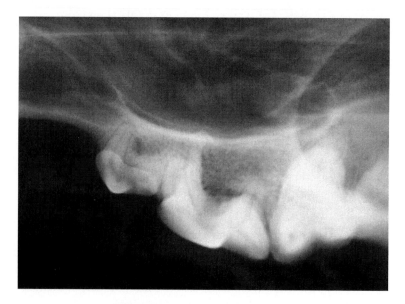

FIGURE 11-15 Foreshortening.

Overlapping Dental Structures

To determine the identity of three-dimensional structures seen on a two-dimensional plane, particularly in the evaluation of maxillary fourth premolar palatal and mesial buccal roots, a second film is taken, with the x-ray beam moved either anterior or posterior to the previous position of the radiographic cone head. The structure that is more lingual (the palatal root) will be shadowed on the film in the same direction as the x-ray beam. The structure that is more buccal (the mesial buccal root) will be shadowed in the opposite direction as the x-ray beam. This phenomenon may be remembered by the acronym "SLOB," which stands for **S**ame **L**ingual **O**pposite **B**uccal. When successive radiographs are taken, the most lingual (palatal) root will move in the same direction on the radiograph as the cone head was repositioned. If the cone is moved forward, the lingual root will be the root that moves forward.

RADIOGRAPHIC FILM PROCESSING

With the standard hand-tank developing method, the same procedure is used as for other x-ray film. Specialized racks or holders may be used to hold the film(s) during the developing process. The advantage of this technique is that additional equipment and material are not required. The most significant disadvantage is the slow developing time. Automatic processors establish constant developing and fixing, eliminating human error and decreasing operator time. Unless the processor is designed to transport small films, this method will present difficulties. Automatic dental film processors are expensive. The use of "leaders" and large film processors is impractical and therefore discouraged. The two-step rapid processing technique is recommended. Solutions designed for rapid developing and fixing of dental film are used in small dip tanks. One tank is for the developer, one or two tanks for the water rinse, and one for the fixer. Small dip tanks may be bought for this purpose or empty, cleaned medicine jars may be used. The dip tanks may be housed in a darkroom or in a "chairside darkroom." A chairside darkroom is a plastic box that allows the developing of radiographs at chairside. The box has two holes for the operator's hands and a plexiglass shield that does not allow the radiograph to be exposed to light but still allows the operator to see the processing.

Technique

The solutions are stirred to mix (Fig. 11-16). In a dark environment the film is opened and attached to a film clip. The film clip must be dry and not contaminated with solution from previous developing radiographs (Fig. 11-17). The paper must be completely removed from the radiographic film or the developer and fixer will not penetrate the paper, and the radiograph will have to be retaken (Fig. 11-18). Placing the film in water for approximately 5 seconds softens the emulsion and ensures equal penetration of the developer into the film.

The film is then immersed in the developer and briefly agitated to remove any bubbles. The time that the film is left in the developer depends on the solution and the temperature; the manufacturer's recommendations should always be followed.

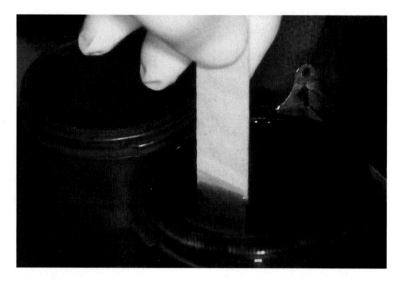

FIGURE 11-16 Mixing radiographic solutions before developing the radiograph. Note that hands are gloved, which should always be the case when working with chemicals.

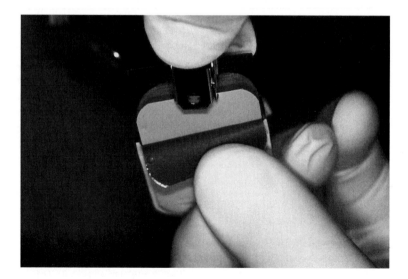

FIGURE 11-17 Placing a clip on the radiographic film to handle the film while developing.

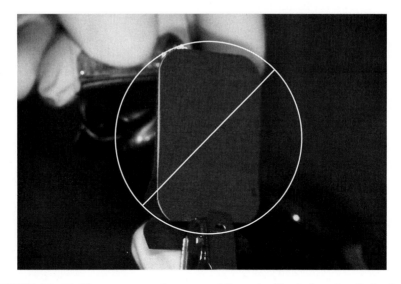

FIGURE 11-18 The paper must be removed from the film before the clip is placed.

The film is removed from the developer with minimal drip-back into the developing tank. The film is placed into the water rinse and dipped five times. The film is then transferred to the fixer and intermittently agitated during its fixing. The fixing is usually twice the developing time.

After the time prescribed by the manufacturer, the film is transferred into the final rinse. The fixer is allowed to drip back into the fixing tank. The film may be read at any time, but it should be returned for a minimum of 10 minutes to a fresh water rinse. (A longer rinse time ensures that all fixer has been removed from the emulsion.)

Developing Complications

Once the film is removed from the protective packet, processing should begin as soon as possible. The following are some complications that can occur during developing.

Clear film

If the film is clear, it has not been exposed to x-ray beams (Fig. 11-19). Failure to turn the radiograph machine on, a burned-out machine tube, and aiming the radiograph machine head incorrectly all can cause this complication.

Light film with poor contrast

If the film is light with poor contrast and other developing problems are eliminated, the film could have been underexposed. Underexposure may be caused by a time setting that was too short, a milliamperage (mA) setting that was too low, or a kilovoltage kV(p) that was too low. Also, the focal-film distance may have been too great.

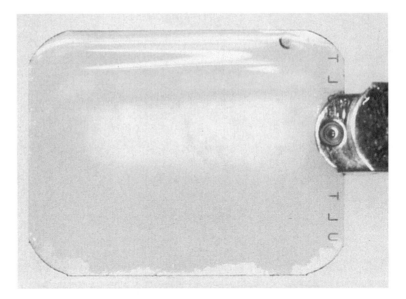

FIGURE 11-19 Clear film that has not been exposed to x-rays.

Finally, the exposure button may have been released prematurely before a full exposure was obtained. Use of old developer causes a washed-out background and fogs the film. If the developing time is too short, a film with low contrast and density will result.

Light film with markings
If cross hatches appear on the film or the image is barely visible and all other aspects of the technique were correct, the problem may be the result of placing the film in the mouth with the wrong side toward the tube head (Fig. 11-20).

Black film
Excessively dark film may be caused by overexposure of the film (Fig. 11-21). Another cause may be a light leak in the darkroom or chairside darkroom (Fig. 11-22). Prolonged viewing of the film between the developing and fixing stage is discouraged; doing so results in an overall grayness of the film.

If Ektaspeed film (EP) is used or the unit is below a bright light source, a red filter should be placed on the amber filter to prevent overexposure. If the film is overdeveloped, excessive density and low contrast will result.

Brown tint
If the film is not fixed sufficiently, it will turn brown with age.

Green tint
Radiographic film that has not been properly rinsed may turn green or splotchy with time. Checking film that was processed several months ago is recommended for quality control.

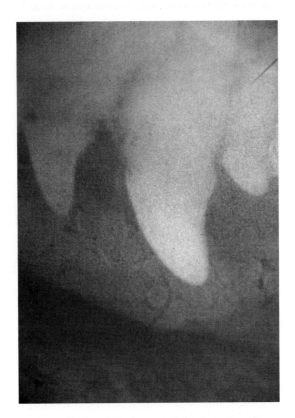

FIGURE 11-20 The film was placed in the mouth backwards and exposed. Note the small circles, which represent indentations in the lead shielding that the x-rays penetrated before exposing the radiographic film.

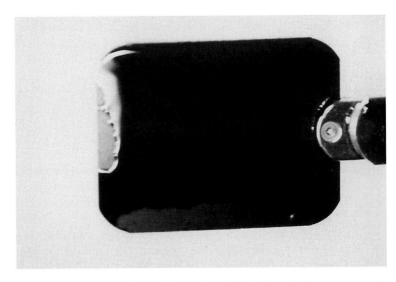

FIGURE 11-21 This film was exposed to light before developing took place.

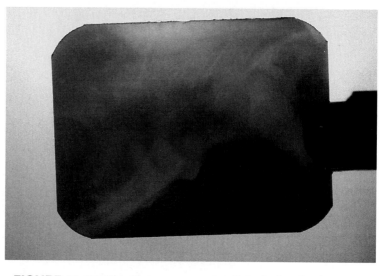

FIGURE 11-22 This film was exposed to light during development.

Solution Disposal

Processing solutions must be discarded in accordance with federal and state guidelines. They should never be poured down the drain.

Film Storage

Envelopes or film mounts can be attached to the patient's medical record (Fig. 11-23). However, this can make the medical record bulky. Often practitioners prefer to store the radiographs separately, either with the larger radiographs taken for other veterinary medical procedures or in a separate file for dental films only.

RADIOGRAPHIC FINDINGS

Normal Young Patient

In the young patient the dentinal wall is thin and the pulp chamber is large. As the tooth develops, odontoblasts that line the pulp chamber produce dentine. Dentine thickens the dentinal wall and reduces the size of the pulp canal. The apex may be open, depending on the age of the patient. In the young patient the dense cortical alveolar bone forming the wall of the socket appears radiographically as a distinct, opaque, uninterrupted, white line parallel to the tooth root. This line is known as the *lamina dura. Lamina dura* is a radiographic term referring to the dense cortical bone forming the wall of the alveolus. The lamina dura appears radiographically as a bony white line next to the dark line of the periodontal space. The radiolucent image between the lamina dura and tooth is the periodontal space and is known as

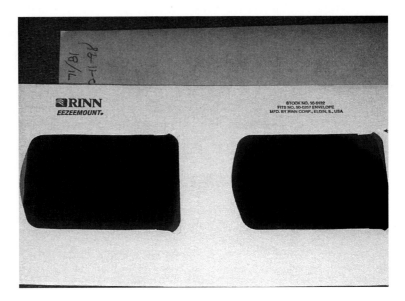

FIGURE 11-23 These radiographs have been placed in film mounts. Later, they will be placed in an envelope for storage.

the *lamina lucida*. It is occupied by the periodontal ligament. The trabecular pattern of interdental bone should also be studied.

Normal Older Patient

The dental radiograph of a healthy adult shows a decreased canal size and increased dentinal wall thickness. Generally, the lamina lucida becomes narrower with age until it disappears. While an apex is present, the apical delta or apical foramen is usually not seen. Thinning of the alveolar crest may occur.

Periodontal Disease

Radiographic signs of periodontal disease include rounding and loss of the alveolar crest. These signs are particularly visible between teeth in the interproximal space, as well as in the furcations. *[Interproximal. The area between adjacent surfaces of adjoining teeth.]* Periodontal disease may also be noted as horizontal bone loss. If vertical bone loss has occurred, increased periodontal ligament space will be evident. Subgingival calculus may be noted (Fig. 11-24).

Endodontic Disease

Signs of endodontic disease include lucency around the apex of the tooth root, resorption of the tooth root internally, or resorption of the tooth root externally (Fig. 11-25). *[Resorption. The loss of substance by a physiologic or pathologic process.]* Fractures may be noted above or below the gumline.

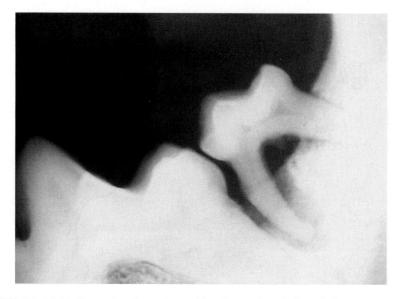

FIGURE 11-24 Radiograph of a patient with advanced periodontal disease; note the extensive bone loss around the mesial root of the mandibular second molar.

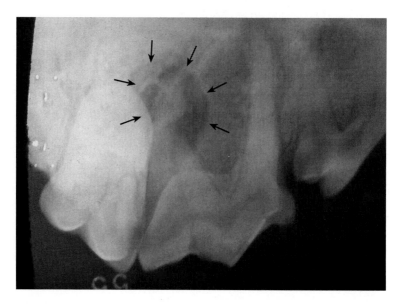

FIGURE 11-25 This radiograph demonstrates a lucency of the bone surrounding the apex of the distal root *(arrows)*.

Cervical Line Lesions

Radiographic signs of a cervical line lesion range from a barely visible coronal lucency to resorption of the entire root. Radiographs should always be taken before filling these lesions (Fig. 11-26).

Retained Roots

Radiographs may be taken, both diagnostically and interoperatively, to evaluate retained roots. The presence of lucency around the root may indicate active infection. The radiograph should be evaluated to determine whether other oral structures have been compromised.

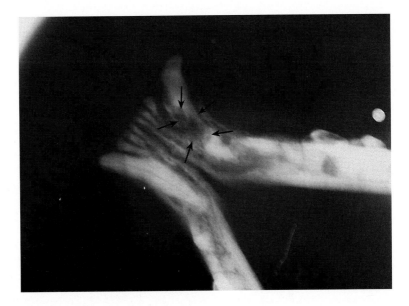

FIGURE 11-26 This radiograph shows a resorptive lesion on the mandibular canine tooth *(arrows)*.

Worksheet

STUDENT NAME: _____

1. Intraoral radiographic film is _____.

2. Most intraoral film is a series of layers. A _____ coating covers the external portion.

3. Between the plastic and the radiographic film itself is a _____ _____ _____.

4. Personnel should be protected by use of _____, _____, and/or safe _____.

5. Dental radiographs can be taken using _____ medical radiographic units.

6. The advantage of the dental radiographic unit is the fairly flexible _____ _____.

7. A maximal amount of _____ and supporting bone should be included in the film.

8. The parallel technique is indicated for radiographs to evaluate _____ _____ _____ and _____ _____.

9. The _____ _____ _____ is used when parallel projections cannot be made.

10. If the radiographic machine is aimed at the tooth, the x-rays will shoot by the film. If anything shows up on the image, it will be distorted by _____.

11. If the radiographic machine is aimed at the film, the x-rays may miss the tooth. A distorted tooth by _____ is the complication with this approach.

12. To radiograph the maxillary posterior teeth, the film is placed in the mouth _____ to the hard palate.

13. To radiograph the maxillary posterior teeth, the radiographic machine head is positioned so that it is _____ degrees off the vertical or horizontal plane of the palate and radiographic film.

14. The complete radiographic study can be obtained in as little as _____ views.

15. The canine teeth are best evaluated by placing the head _____ degrees from the front of the patient and _____ degrees from the side of the patient.

16. Blurred or double images are caused by _____ of either the patient of the x-ray machine head.

17. _____ film is film that has been overexposed, overdeveloped, or exposed to light during processing.

18. _____ film is film that has not been exposed to x-rays.

19. Old _____ gives a washed-out background and fogs the film.

20. Processing solutions should never be poured down the _____.

12

Advanced Veterinary Dental Procedures

Periodontal Surgery, Endodontics, Restorations and Orthodontics

At one time, veterinary dentistry meant either scraping calculus from the teeth or extracting them if they could not be saved by conservative techniques. Fortunately for the patient, dentistry has made significant advances. Although not all practices have the resources to perform advanced procedures, the veterinary staff should have an idea of the range of procedures that can be performed to save teeth, what each procedure entails, and the type of equipment necessary. Some practices may perform many advanced dental procedures, and this chapter briefly addresses the most common. For a more detailed discussion, texts such as *Veterinary Dental Techniques* (W.B. Saunders); *Veterinary Dentistry, Principles and Practice* (Lippincott-Raven); and *Small Animal Dentistry* (Mosby) should be consulted.

PERIODONTAL SURGICAL TECHNIQUES

Periodontal surgical techniques are employed after more conservative measures, such as closed periodontal debridement, have been attempted without success or have been ruled out as impossible. In periodontal surgery, flaps are created to expose the tooth root and associated bone. The bone may be reshaped or augmented, and the gingiva may be sutured back to the initial position. Alternatively, the gingival height may be changed apically by gingival or bone surgery to decrease the pocket or coronally with guided tissue regeneration to increase the height of attachment.

Evaluation for Procedure

A periodontal probe and dental radiographs are used diagnostically before the procedure to determine the location of the pocket and to aid in the selection of an appropriate form of therapy.

Goal of Periodontal Surgery

The goal of periodontal surgery is to eliminate pockets harboring subgingival plaque and calculus. The ultimate aim is to prevent subgingival plaque and calculus from returning.

Instruments and Materials

Periodontal surgery requires various instruments and materials (Box 12-1). The No. 3 handle is the standard type for scalpels. A variety of different blades may be used, including special periodontal knives. The No.15c blade is extremely fine and therefore useful in periodontal surgical procedures. In addition, small tissue scissors, such as LaGrange scissors, are helpful in trimming periodontal tissue. Periosteal elevators are used to lift the gingiva away from the bone. Several types are available. The Molt elevator is one type, the Molt No.9 being particularly popular. Many practitioners also like the ST-No.7 instruments. Having a variety of periodontal surgical instruments available makes treating various anatomic and pathologic conditions less difficult.

Solutions for irrigating the tissue are also important in periodontal surgery. Sterile saline solution and chlorhexidine are most common. Chlorhexidine is used in a 0.1% to 0.2% solution and is available in two forms: diacetate and gluconate. Gluconate is preferred.

Tissue forceps and needle holders are necessary for suturing. Although expensive, the best is the spring-locking Castroviejo-type needle holder. For the sutures themselves, 4-0 or 5-0 absorbable material with a reverse cutting FS-2 needle is used. The high-speed handpiece is used in the removal of bone, and burs may be added for the removal of granulation tissue. Round burs (#2 or #4), crosscut fissure burs (#701L), or pear-shaped burs (#330) may be used in the appropriate handpiece. Bone files may be used to contour bone.

BOX 12-1
Instruments and Materials for Periodontal Surgery

No. 3 (or similar) scalpel handle
15c scalpel blades
Small tissue scissors (LaGrange)
Periosteal elevator: Molt (No.2, No.4, or No.9), ST-No.7
Scaling curette
Sterile saline solution
Chlorhexidine 0.1 to 0.2% diacetate or gluconate (gluconate preferred)
Tissue forceps
Needle holders, spring locking (Castroviejo)
4-0 or 5-0 absorbable or nonabsorbable suture material with reverse FS-2 cutting needle
High-speed handpiece
#2 or #4 round burs, appropriate for handpiece used
Bone files

Treatment Techniques

Hyperplastic gingiva

Because gingivoplasty (gingivectomy) is performed only when hyperplastic gingiva is present, patients must be selected carefully. Gingivoplasty should not be used for treatment of deep periodontal pockets or as part of the routine prophy. This procedure is contraindicated when attached gingiva is minimal or absent or horizontal or vertical bone loss is present below the mucogingival junction. *[Mucogingival junction. The line of demarcation where the attached gingiva and alveolar mucosa meet.]* These characteristics are prevalent in certain breeds and breed lines, particularly boxers and collies.

Gingivoplasty technique

The pocket depth and contour is determined by inserting a probe to the depth of the pocket at several areas around the tooth. The corresponding depth is measured on the outside of the gingiva, also using the probe. A bleeding point is made by placing the tip of the probe perpendicular to the gingiva and applying slight pressure to make a small hole or by using a small-gauge needle. Bleeding points are made around the contour of the pocket and are used as a guide for the gingivectomy. The gingivectomy is made at an angle apical to the bleeding point to create a beveled margin. At least 2 mm of healthy, attached gingiva must be present apical to the base of the incision. A scalpel blade or electrosurgery blade is used to excise the gingiva by cutting below the bleeding points, with the blade held at approximately a 45-degree angle and the tip of the blade toward the crown. The ends of the excision should be tapered into the surrounding gingiva to create the normal scalloped contour, particularly if several adjacent teeth are treated. Gingival tags can be removed with the blade or a sharp curette. The exposed tooth and root surface can now be scaled and planed smooth. Hemorrhage is controlled by applying pressure with wet gauze pads or hemostatic agents. If electrosurgery is being performed, caution must be exercised because the collateral damage may extend past the desired surgical line. In Fig. 12-1 a periodontal probe is used to measure the pocket and a scalpel blade is used to perform the gingivoplasty.

Deep periodontal pocket

Treatment of deep periodontal pockets beyond the range of closed periodontal debridement requires either extraction of the tooth or creation of a periodontal flap and treatment. The flap allows visualization of subgingival tissues. By creating a flap and reflecting the periodontal tissues off the tooth surface, the practitioner can see the tooth surface where periodontal debridement or root planing is being performed.

Indications for open flap and root planing

Generally, it is best to attempt the more conservative treatment of closed periodontal debridement before performing open surgery, if the pocket is greater than 5 mm in depth. After the flap is created, periodontal debridement or root planing is performed.

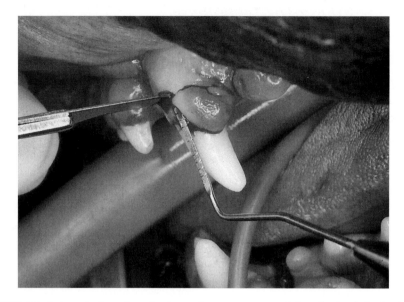

FIGURE 12-1 A periodontal probe is used to measure, and the gingiva is incised with a scalpel.

Open flap and root planing technique

The gingiva is disinfected. An incision should be made that follows the contour of the tooth running in the sulcus. Releasing incisions are created, starting at the line angle of the teeth mesial and distal to the surgery site. The gingiva is elevated with the periosteal elevator lingually/palatally and labially/buccally without exposing the marginal alveolar bone. The exposed root surfaces are planed until they are smooth and hard. Before closure the area is flushed with chlorhexidine solution. The flap is repositioned and sutured with interrupted sutures placed interdentally.

Excessive attachment of frenula

Dogs have two mandibular frenula, located distal to the mandibular canine teeth. Although these frenula help hold the lower lip close to the gums, they may be too tight in some patients. Excessive tightness allows an accumulation of debris on the distal side of the canine teeth. The frenoplasty procedure is designed to loosen the lip from the gingiva (Fig. 12-2).

A mandibular frenoplasty (frenectomy) is indicated in patients with gingival recession or pocket formation on the distal side of the canine teeth caused by the presence of the frenulum. The objective of the procedure is to minimize the accumulation of food in the anterior portion of the mouth and improve self-cleansing of this area.

The attachment of the frenulum to the mandibular gingiva near the first premolar is cut horizontally with scissors or a blade. The cut is extended into the frenulum to release the pull of the muscular attachments with the blade or scissors. The lip relaxes laterally when the attachments have been completely cut. The cut surfaces create a diamond shape. Suturing brings the mesial and distal edges together. Several simple

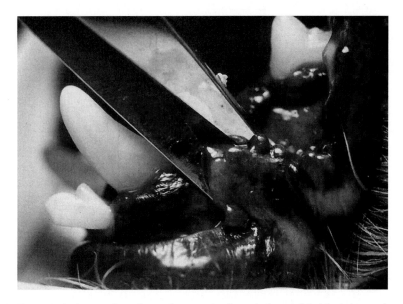

FIGURE 12-2 A sharp scissor is used to cut the frenula located behind the canine teeth.

interrupted sutures of an absorbable material are placed to prevent reattachment. The root surfaces of the canines should be planed smooth and polished.

Oronasal fistula

Three techniques are used in oronasal fistula (ONF) repair. *[Oronasal fistula. An abnormal opening between the oral and nasal cavities.]* These are the simple sliding flap, the double palatal/sliding flap, and the double palatal/pedicle flap. All are variations of the same procedure.

The simple buccal sliding flap is usually used for smaller fistulas. If the fistula is large or chronic, a double palatal/sliding flap is recommended. The margins of the fistula are debrided of necrotic and epithelialized tissue. The alveolar bone may require recontouring to allow better positioning of the flap. Recontouring is accomplished with a small rongeur, chisel, or curette. The flap is sutured with 3-0 or 4-0 sutures. If the simple flap fails, a variety of advanced flaps can be placed.

Follow-up Recommendations for All Periodontal Surgery

After surgery the patient should be given a soft diet for 1 to 7 days. Oral antibiotics are administered as appropriate. The oral cavity is flushed with chlorhexidine solution for 2 weeks. After the patient's wounds have healed, oral hygiene should be performed in the home to minimize future plaque accumulations.

After the surgical site has healed, home care must be continued. The product selected for use depends on the patient's particular situation. Postsurgical checkups are important to monitor the patient's progress. A minimum of two follow-up appointments should be scheduled for 10 days and 1 month after the procedure. Additional appointments may be scheduled if necessary. Because patients that have had periodontal surgery sometimes experience a relapse, monthly or quarterly follow-up visits may be necessary.

ENDODONTICS AND RESTORATIONS

At one time, veterinarians did not treat fractured teeth. Consequently, many patients suffered silently as the tooth first died and then became abscessed. Endodontic therapy is a better option. *Endodontic therapy* is a general term for treatment of the dental pulp and may be used to save vital pulp, remove live or dead pulp, and prevent or treat infection.

Pulp tissue consists of blood vessels, nerves, and connective tissues that support the odontoblastic cells lining the pulp chamber and root canal. Throughout life the odontoblasts produce dentine that fills in the canal. As a result, the dentine layer thickens with age.

Bacteria usually gain entry to the pulp chamber via a fractured tooth. The pulpal tissue becomes inflamed and edematous and dies. Then bacteria move into the apical region of the tooth. From this area, they spread through the canals in the apical delta of the tooth, which formerly served as tunnels for the nerves and blood vessels. Once the bacteria enter the apical bone, an abscess starts. The periapical abscess may eventually (i.e., years later) become walled off, cause inflammatory resorption of the root, spread along the periodontal ligament, and cause ankylosis (fusion) of the tooth root with the surrounding bone.

Discolored teeth, especially those that are pink and purple, indicate pulpal hemorrhage and necessitate root canal therapy. Caution should be exercised in young animals because the tooth may be discolored as a result of trauma yet retain sufficient blood supply to survive and continue to develop. If a root canal is performed on this type of tooth and the tooth walls are not completely developed, the tooth may fracture. In young patients, evaluation through radiography is advised.

Indications for Endodontic Therapy

The most common indication for root canal therapy is fractured teeth. If the tip of the crown appears black, the patient is a candidate for a workup and evaluation of the tooth. Cats are particularly susceptible to canine tooth abscess. The pulp chamber extends close to the tip, and any exposure of dentine allows bacteria into the pulp chamber. Chronic abscess of the canine teeth is extremely common in cats; all fractured teeth necessitate root canal therapy, extraction, or close monitoring.

A worn tooth with a brown covering in the area where the pulp chamber used to be indicates that the wear has occurred slowly enough that secondary dentine was deposited by the odontoblasts lining the root canal and pulp chamber. In this case, the tooth should be evaluated radiographically. Occasionally, teeth that are completely normal in appearance may have apical disease that can be diagnosed only radiographically.

The rationale for endodontic treatment is to maintain optimal health. A tooth with endodontic disease produces various signs, including pain and irritability. Many patients with endodontic disease exhibit fluctuations in appetite. Clients frequently report halitosis, or bad breath, in pets with undiagnosed endodontic disease.

Once pulpal death occurs, most dogs and cats do not show pain. However, if the tooth is alive and recently traumatized, many patients flinch when the tooth is percussed with a probe or other instrument. Some animals chew food only on the side of the mouth opposite to the traumatized tooth, or they drool and produce increased calculus on the injured side. Hunting dogs may refuse their training dummies, utility dogs may refuse their dumbbells, and attack dogs may either hesitate or bite and release repetitively because of the pain (this is referred to as *typewriting*). Dogs that are used for tracking scents may be less effective than usual because of the odor from the oral infection, which overwhelms the scent.

When pulp exposure is secondary to a coronal fracture or a carious erosion, pathogenic bacteria soon descend into the pulp canal and cause an abscess either within the canal itself or periapically by extension of the infection. Infection that has penetrated the apical end of the root canal can cause osteomyelitis and the subsequent loss of surrounding bone. Periapical infection can spread, contributing to pathologic fractures of the lower jaw, or the infection can extend through weakened necrotic bone and develop into an oronasal fistula from any of the maxillary teeth (Fig. 12-3).

Advantage of Endodontic Therapy

Endodontic therapy is much less invasive than surgical extraction of a large canine *[Canine tooth. Large, single-rooted tooth designed for puncturing, tearing, and grasping.]* or

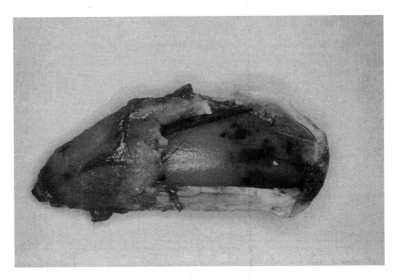

FIGURE 12-3 This patient's tooth was fractured. The client was advised to ignore it. Within 8 months, extraction was necessary. Note the foreign material (foxtail) that found its way into the exposed pulp chamber.

carnassial tooth *[Carnassial tooth. Shearing tooth. Upper P4 and lower M1 in the dog and cat.]*; it can therefore be performed more easily and quickly than a surgical procedure. Standard root canal therapy is less traumatic for the patient and more aesthetically pleasing to the owner than surgical extraction. Moreover, the cost of root canal therapy is equivalent to that of surgical extraction. Another advantage of small animal endodontics is that a well-done procedure is less likely to fail in the pet's lifetime because the patient has a relatively short life span.

Endodontic Procedures

Vital pulpotomy

Vital pulpotomy is indicated for recent fractures to preserve healthy dental pulp. This procedure should be performed within 48 hours of the fracture of a mature tooth. In an incompletely developed adult tooth, this time can be extended to 2 or 3 weeks after the fracture. In such a case, the young tooth will ideally develop a thicker and stronger dentinal wall during the extended time period, even if persistent infection later necessitates standard root canal therapy.

A vital pulpotomy is performed by removing the exposed, contaminated pulp and gently disinfecting the remaining pulp and access site. Calcium hydroxide is applied to stimulate the formation of a dentinal bridge, and a strong base interface is installed to support the surface restoration material of metal or a composite.

Direct pulp-capping

Direct pulp-capping resembles vital pulpotomy but is performed after purposeful or accidental iatrogenic pulpal exposure. The pulp may be intentionally exposed during a disarming procedure in which all four canines are coronally reduced to the level of the adjacent incisors. This procedure may also be performed on one or two maloccluded mandibular canines to relieve traumatic penetration of the upper gingiva or palate. This procedure is performed aseptically. The materials installed are the same as those used in a vital pulpotomy. The pulp does not require disinfecting, however, because the teeth are invaded in a sterile manner.

Indirect pulp-capping

Indirect pulp-capping is a restorative procedure performed when the preparation of a carious lesion does not penetrate the pulp but is perilously close (0.5 mm) to it. For such incidences, a therapeutic and insulating base layer of quick-setting calcium hydroxide paste is installed to protect the pulp. It is followed by the preparation for and the installation of an appropriate surface restoration.

Standard Root Canal Therapy

Standard root canal therapy (formerly called *conventional root canal therapy*) is also known as *pulpectomy*. In this procedure the pulp canal is approached in a normograde direction (from the crown to the apex). The entire pulp is removed through either the fracture site or one or more drilled access holes.

Standard root canal therapy is indicated for adult teeth that are discolored and endodontically dead or contaminated with long-standing infection. In a mature tooth a long-standing infection is one in which the pulp has been contaminated for more than 48 hours. In an immature tooth, long-standing infection means that the pulp has been contaminated for more than 2 weeks.

Endodontic Equipment

Endodontic therapy requires various instruments and materials (Box 12-2). The equipment required includes barbed broaches, reamers, files, irrigating needles, mixing slab (or paper pad), spatula, pluggers, and spreaders (Fig. 12-4). Materials are discussed in more detail later in this chapter.

Barbed broaches

A barbed broach (Fig. 12-5) is manufactured by making deep incisions in a soft iron wire, creating flared barbs. This instrument is not strong, but it is useful in removing intact pulp. The broach can also be used to remove from the root canal absorbent points, cotton pellets, separated file tips, and other foreign material, such as dirt, gravel, and grass.

Files and reamers

Files and reamers are used to clean the canal and remove dead or infected tissues (Fig. 12-6). Reamers are an earlier style of file but are still preferred by some practi-

---

BOX 12-2
Endodontic Equipment, Instruments, and Materials

Cutting bur: tapered cross-cut fissure burs #170L, round burs #2, #4, pear-shaped burs #330
Barbed broaches
K-files & Hedström files: Numbers 06, 08, 10, 15, 20, 25, 30, 35, 40, 45, 50, 55, 60, 70, 80, 90, 100 in 31 and 45 mm (minimum—longer files may be necessary)
Endodontic stops
Endodontic rings
Irrigation needles
Mixing slab and spatula
RC-Prep
Canal irrigant: sodium hypochlorite, chlorhexidine
Paper absorbent points: similar size to files
Root canal sealer: ZOE or advanced sealers
Gutta-percha
Endodontic point forceps: cotton or college pliers
Pluggers and spreaders: short and long length
Restorative materials
Finishing disks, points, or stones

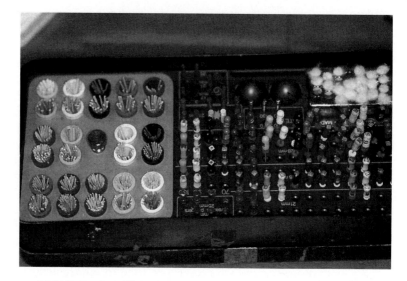

FIGURE 12-4 This tray provides compact storage for materials.

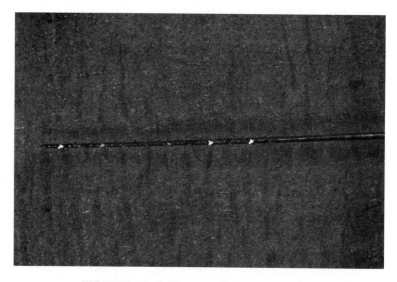

FIGURE 12-5 Close up of a barbed broach.

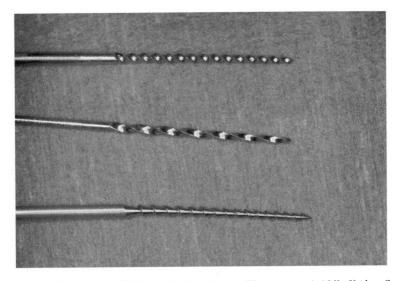

FIGURE 12-6 K-file *(upper file)* has fairly tight flutes. The reamer *(middle file)* has flutes that are more widely spaced. The Hedström file *(lower file)* has sharper flutes than the K-file or reamer. These styles are manufactured for different distributors and can be purchased in premium or economy grades.

tioners. They are twisted, square metal rods with fewer flutes (or twists) per millimeter than on a file. Reamers are used in a twisting, augerlike motion that delivers filings from the depth of the canal to the access site.

The K-files are stiffer and stronger, size for size, than the Hedström files because of the way they are manufactured. To create K-files, a square, rhomboid, or triangular rod is twisted, creating cutting flutes. The K-file is similar in design to a reamer but has a tighter twist and is operated either by making a push-and-pull motion or by rotating clockwise 90 degrees and pulling coronally. It will break easily if is lodged tightly in the canal and then twisted counterclockwise in an effort to dislodge it. K-files produce a clean, smooth canal wall and, because of their design, are best used to cleanse and shape the apical portion of the canal.

A Hedström file is created when a spiral groove is machined into the rod. It is weaker than a K-file because its core has been reduced in diameter by the machine. The shape of a Hedström file is that of inner-stacked cones. Its carrier effect is produced by a straight pull of the file. Hedström files produce a clean, but not cylindrical or smooth, wall. They are used to cleanse and shape the coronal or incisal portion of the canal.

Files and reamers have two dimensions, length and diameter. A millimeter (mm) notation indicates the length. Usually two lengths are needed, 25 mm and 31 mm for incisors, premolars, and molars and 45 mm and 60 mm for canines (Fig. 12-7). The diameter is indicated by a number only, which represents the diameter of the file at the working end. A No. 10 file is 0.1 mm at the working end, and a No. 100 file is 1.0

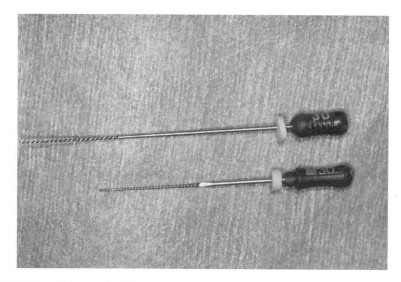

FIGURE 12-7 These are both No. 30 files; the upper file is 45 mm in length, and the lower file is 31 mm in length.

mm at the working end. Files are stored in endodontic organizers. As they are pulled out and used, they may be stored (and cleaned) intraoperatively with an Endo-ring, which has an attached sponge and ruler. Before they are placed in the organizer, the files are cleaned and disinfected or sterilized.

Files and reamers are color coded to identify them by size. The numbers are repeated, however, so caution is necessary to prevent files of similar color but different size from being confused. The color-coding system is as follows:

Grey: 08
Purple: 10
White: 15, 45, 90, 150
Yellow: 20, 50, 100
Red: 25, 55, 110
Blue: 30, 60, 120
Green: 35, 70, 130
Black: 40, 80, 140

Newer types of files are available that increase by a percentage rather than by 0.05 mm or 0.1 mm. These files have their own color-coding system, which must be identified by the manufacturer.

Because an endodontic file is a cutting instrument, it operates most efficiently when sharp. The smaller sizes are delicate and prone to bending. They may also unravel, manifested by a shiny area between two cutting flutes, with repeated or improper use. Breakage occurs soon after a file has begun to unravel or after a file has been bent and subsequently straightened by the clinician (Fig. 12-8).

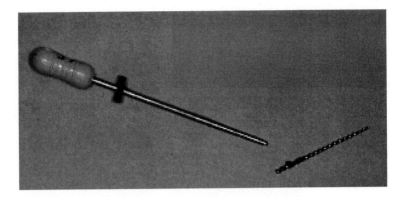

FIGURE 12-8 Fractured K-file. The tip of the file was removed from the canal by using ultrasonic vibration.

Endodontic stops

Endodontic stops are pieces of rubber material placed on the file or reamer to aid in marking the length of the instrument. To find the apical working depth, smaller files are placed in the canal, the stop is moved to the point where the file has entered the tooth, and a radiograph is taken. Once evaluated, the placement of the stop is adjusted so that the tip of the file reaches the apex when the stop just touches the access point. This distance is also measured.

Endo-ring

An Endo-ring is a metal or plastic instrument that fits around the finger (Fig. 12-9). An attached disposable sponge, in which the files can be placed in ascending order of size, helps organize the files during the procedure. In addition, the sponge helps clean the files during the endodontic procedure.

Irrigation materials

Irrigating solutions are introduced into the canal by means of a 27-gauge, blunt-tipped endodontic needle. Sodium hypochlorite helps break down and remove the organic material. When a file is being exchanged for a larger file (or whenever the canal is thought dry), the canal is flushed with a 1.5% sodium hypochlorite solution. This solution is made by mixing 1 part sodium hypochlorite to 3 parts water. RC Prep® is an EDTA chelating agent. This helps break down the inorganic material. A final flush is made with sodium hypochlorite.

Endodontic materials

Absorbent points are used for drying the pulp canal after it has been prepared (debrided) and irrigated. Absorbent points are tightly rolled, tapered paper available in sizes 15 to 80, which correspond to file sizes. They are available in lengths of 30 mm and 55 mm. Absorbent points are disposable. Each size can be purchased in lots of

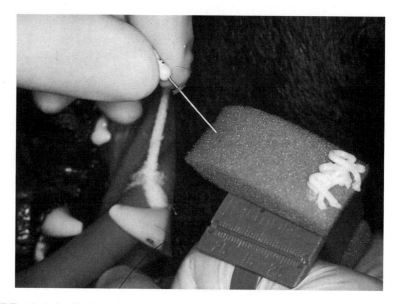

FIGURE 12-9 An Endo-ring. The material on the right side of the sponge is RC Prep, an agent used to break down the inorganic portion of the tooth.

200 or fewer points, or they can be ordered in assorted sizes in conveniently organized packages. It is best to keep both lengths in every size on hand.

The root canal is sealed to prevent bacteria from entering the canal. Cements or pastes are used to seal the apical one-third of the root, dentinal tubules that radiate from the walls of the canal, and apical delta. *[Lateral or accessory canal. The small canal branching from the root canal to the outer surface of the root, usually occurring in the apical third of the root.]* There are several categories of root canal sealants, but two types are used most often in veterinary medicine. The first is a eugenol-based sealant, ZOE. Used commonly in standard root canal procedures, it is best known for providing a long working time and being a good, nonirritating antimicrobial agent. Some dentists criticize it as being a temporary sealant because ZOE cements disintegrate after 5 to 8 years in the oral cavity. For most purposes, however, it is quite adequate for veterinary use because the life span of a dog or cat is much shorter than that of a person. The sealer is mixed by a figure-eight mixing motion.

Mixing should be performed on a glass slab or paper mixing pad. Zinc oxide and eugenol (ZOE) are combined. The proper consistency is obtained when the ZOE sticks to the spatula for a distance of ½ to 1 inch off the mixing pad (Fig. 12-10). Zinc oxide/eugenol may be placed on the gutta-percha point and then carried into the canal with the gutta-percha. This method works well with small (up to No. 30) canals.

Gutta-percha is the most popular core material used by veterinary practitioners. It does not irritate the periapical tissues and is highly condensable. It is used to help remove voids in the canal sealer and provide a better seal of the apex and openings

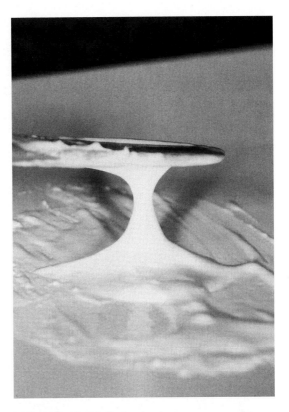

FIGURE 12-10 Seal mixed to proper consistency whereby the material spans the spatula and pad by approximately one-half inch before separating.

to the dentinal tubules that radiate from the walls of the canal. Gutta-percha points, like absorbent points, are supplied in sizes 15 to 100 and in lengths of 30 mm and 55 mm to correspond with file sizes. Gutta-percha is harvested from a rubber-type tree and is more commonly used in the softened beta form, which is more flexible and less brittle than the natural alpha form. Distributed to the clinician in the beta form, the material transforms to the less flexible and more brittle alpha form as its shelf life expires.

Pluggers

A plugger is used to obtain vertical (apical) condensation. Pluggers have blunted tips (Fig. 12-11). They are used to vertically compact gutta-percha. Various lengths and diameters are available, including those specially designed for veterinary medicine.

Spreaders have a tapered, round shaft with a pointed tip. They are used to compress gutta-percha laterally and force sealant into dentinal tubules. By spreading the gutta-percha laterally, they make room for additional gutta-percha. Combination plugger-spreaders are available. Compared with the plugger, the spreader has a pointed tip (Fig. 12-12).

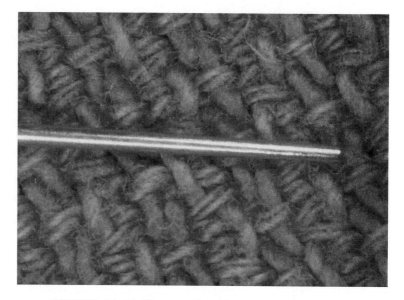

FIGURE 12-11 Close up of a plugger (note the blunt tip).

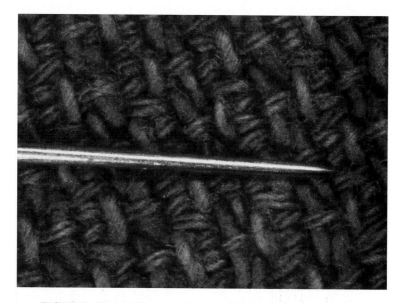

FIGURE 12-12 Close up of a spreader (note the pointed tip).

Endodontic Technique

The following steps are performed in conventional, nonsurgical root canal therapy:
1. Evaluate the need for the procedure
2. Expose the pulp chamber/root canal
3. File and clean the canal
4. Fill the canal with gutta-percha
5. Prepare and fill the access site and any exposed fracture site

Radiographs

Radiographs must be taken throughout the entire endodontic procedure. They are taken initially for diagnostic purposes. In the initial filing a small rubber marker is placed on the file before insertion into the canal. The tooth is radiographed, which allows the practitioner to evaluate the length of the canal. When final filing of the canal is nearly complete, radiographs help the practitioner determine the depth and width of the filing procedure. After the canal has been filled, radiographs help the practitioner evaluate the seal and fill of the canal (Fig. 12-13). If an apical seal is not obtained, the gutta-percha should be either condensed to seal or removed and the filling started over again.

Apicoectomy

Apicoectomy (retrograde or surgical) root canal therapy is indicated for peracute pulpal infections and as a treatment after standard root canal therapy has failed. It

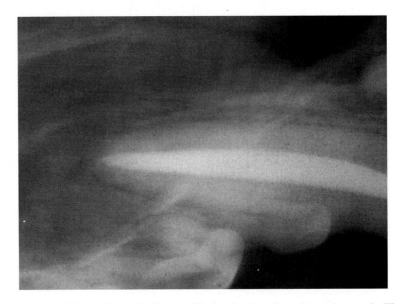

FIGURE 12-13 This radiograph shows a filled pulp chamber of a canine tooth. The sealer and gutta-percha are radiodense, so they appear on the radiograph.

is also indicated when standard treatment presents anatomic or mechanical problems that prevent the completion of an adequate seal of the apical one-third of the root canal.

After standard root canal therapy, apicoectomy is performed on adult teeth in dogs and cats by approaching the apex of the root surgically through the alveolus. This procedure is rarely required in small animals, but it is highly successful in treating difficult cases in which greater access and visibility are required.

RESTORATIVE DENTISTRY

Four types of dental restoratives are available to protect a tooth after endodontic treatment. The best material for the procedure depends on the desired appearance and the amount of trauma the tooth will be subjected to in the future. The purpose of restorative dentistry is to restore the form and function of damaged teeth.

Surface defects, whether iatrogenic (e.g., from drilling into a tooth) or caused by fracture, should be filled with a restorative material to protect the deeper filling materials used in treating the tooth. The cause of fractured and nonvital teeth is usually occlusal trauma, which occurs when the mandibular teeth strike the maxillary teeth or when an object is caught between the upper and lower teeth. This trauma can occur, for example, when a dog plays Frisbee or chews on objects harder than the teeth or when external forces are directed against the teeth. In most cases the patient will subject its teeth to further trauma after the tooth has been treated. A restoration protects the integrity of the crown and returns the tooth to its previous form and function. The restoration must be confluent with the margin of the defect and have the smoothest surface possible; this delays the formation of plaque and calculus on the surface of the restoration and prevents moisture leakage at its margins.

Four types of restoratives are commonly used in veterinary dentistry:
- Amalgam (silver alloys)
- Composites (plastics)
- Class II glass ionomers
- Full coverage metal or porcelain-fused-to-metal crowns

Amalgam Restoration

Of the restoratives, amalgam withstands the greatest compressive force but is the least cosmetically appealing. It is usually used to fill defects on the occlusal surface of molars in dogs and of canine cusps of service dogs.

Amalgam is the hardest of the surface restoratives. It has been used since the 1800s and is the easiest to install of the dental restorative materials. Amalgam is the most consistently successful and most convenient to use when purchased in prepared capsules containing a protective membrane between the amalgam alloy and mercury. In capsule form, this material is safer for chairside assistants and the clinician because the fingers have less contact with the mercury. Amalgam is usually reserved for use either on the occlusal surfaces of the posterior teeth in pet dogs or in the anterior *[Anterior teeth. The canine and incisor teeth.]* and posterior teeth *[Posterior teeth. The premolar and molar teeth.]* of service dogs. The disadvantages of amalgam are as follows:

1. Traditionally, amalgam is held in place entirely mechanically and requires a greater undercut preparation than composites or glass ionomers. Making a greater undercut structurally weakens smaller teeth. However, agents that bond amalgam to tooth structure have recently become available.

2. Although amalgam is considered self-sealing, the process is corrosive. When the seal is complete, the margin of the restoration is seen as a black corrosive line (Fig. 12-14).

Composite Restoration

Composites are second only to amalgam in hardness and are more aesthetically pleasing. Composites are installed on the rostral teeth and premolars. They must be applied in a dry environment. Composites are the most commonly used class of restorative material in veterinary dentistry. The use of light-cure composite restorations is recommended. Composites used in veterinary dentistry, like other dental restoratives, are manufactured for use in humans. However, dogs have a bite that is three times as powerful as that of humans. Dogs also abuse their teeth more than humans do.

The restoration site is prepared using a bur of the appropriate size and shape. As little of the tooth structure is removed as possible to prevent weakening but still allow for a macromechanical bond (mechanical retention) with the restorative material.

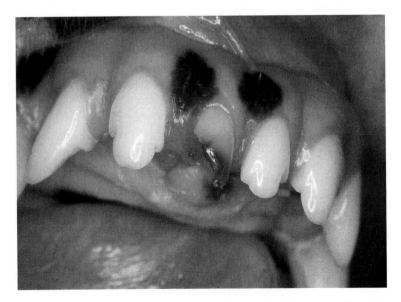

FIGURE 12-14 An amalgam restoration several years after placement. Note the staining.

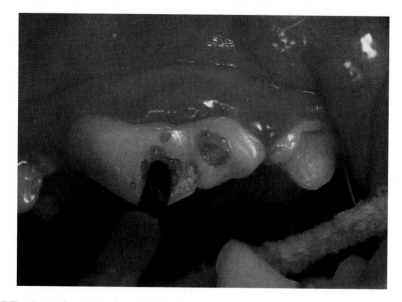

FIGURE 12-15 An acid etch gel is placed on this tooth before placement of the restoration.

The site is cleaned with flour pumice to remove any surface oils that would interfere with adhesion to the composite resin. The pumice, which is commercially available, is a highly siliceous material of volcanic origin. It should be mixed with oil-free (filtered) water until it reaches the consistency of a thick paste. Composites do not cure in a moist environment, such as blood, saliva, or water. Even the oil from the operator's fingertips or contaminated water or air sprays will negatively affect the setting properties of composite resin. Blood also stains uncured composite. The site must be rinsed to remove the pumice residue and then air-dried.

A conditioner/etchant, which is an acid, is applied with a disposable brush to remove the powdered tooth debris (smear layer), 1 to 5 microns thick, created by the cutting bur. The conditioner makes tiny etches in the tooth's surface. Etching permits bonding agents to later penetrate into the etch-induced micro-irregularities and thereby form interlocking tags (Fig. 12-15).

The bonding agents are a primer and an adhesive. The primer, a chemical that tolerates moisture, is applied with a disposable brush (Fig. 12-16). The surface may be slightly damp. The primer should be allowed to set according to the manufacturer's recommendation (usually 5 to 60 seconds) and then blotted or air-dried (depending on the product). The primer fills the microetched surface and prepares it for bonding.

After the primer has been applied, a thin layer of adhesive should be applied with another disposable brush. The adhesive itself has little strength. The composite supplies strength to the restoration. In some bonding products, the primer and adhesive are combined. Adhesives may be either chemically activated or light activated, depending on the product.

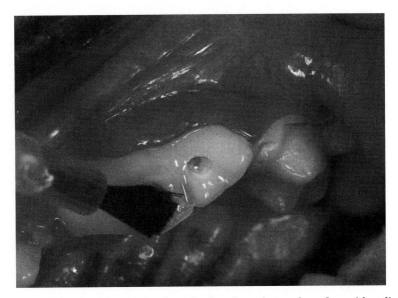

FIGURE 12-16 A bonding agent primer is placed on the tooth surface with a disposable brush.

Finally, the defect is filled with composite, leaving no voids. First, a layer of composite no more than 2 mm to 3 mm thick is applied (Fig. 12-17). This layer is light cured for 40 to 60 seconds, according to the manufacturer's instructions. Layering continues in this manner until the defect is slightly overfilled and the composite overlaps the margins of the defect.

The restored tooth is finished, or smoothed, until its surface is shiny and flawless. Finishing methods vary and include the use of the following instruments:

1. A fine garnet, followed by an extra-fine sandpaper abrasive disc on a low-speed contra angle
2. A composite finishing green stone followed by a white Arkansas stone bur (Fig. 12-18) on a low- or high-speed handpiece
3. 12-, 16-, and then 30-fluted finishing burs. Finishing disks work best for fairly flat, broad surfaces. Rotating stones are useful when working close to the gingival margin or when recreating a developmental groove in the tooth's surface.

Glass Ionomer Restorations

Glass ionomers are not as strong as amalgam and plastics, but bond very well with dentine, deliver fluoride to the dentinal wall, and do not shrink. Glass ionomers do not require an absolutely moisture-free installation site. When the restoration will be subjected to abrasive forces, ionomers can be used as an adherent base beneath a composite, which can better withstand these forces. Glass ionomers are best suited to fill defects in nonocclusal surfaces. However, because of the limited chewing habits of domestic cats, glass ionomers are well suited to fill the access sites in the cusps of

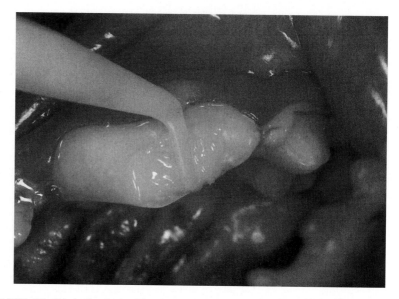

FIGURE 12-17 A plastic working instrument is used to place the composite material.

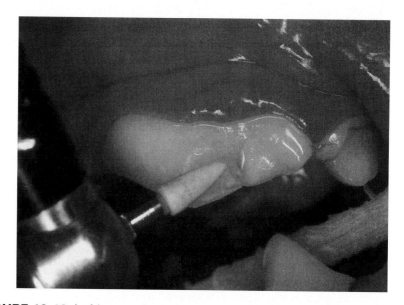

FIGURE 12-18 A white stone is used to shape and smooth the cured composite resin.

the feline canine tooth. They are particularly useful for small teeth because they bond well with dentine and therefore require minimal surface preparation. Glass ionomers are more compatible with the tooth than composites and amalgam, which are more susceptible to expansion and contraction. In addition, glass ionomers contain fluoride.

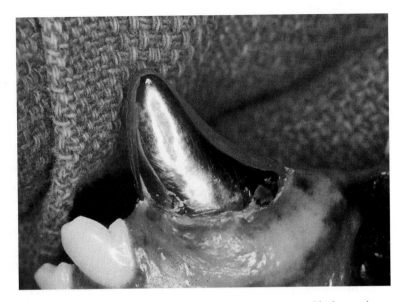

FIGURE 12-19 This crown has been placed on the left mandibular canine tooth.

After the area has been shaped, the restoration site is prepared with a mixture of flour pumice and water. The tooth is rinsed and air-dried. A mild conditioner (poly-acrylic acid) is applied to the restoration site to remove the smear layer. The glass ionomer restorative (mixed according to manufacturer's instructions if it is a two-part product) is placed into the defect, with special effort made to eliminate any voids or air bubbles in the restoration. A Centrix syringe, jiffy tube, or a discoid ex-cavator can be used. Glass ionomers have the least wear resistance of all the com-monly used restorative materials. They do, however, bond well to dentine and, to a certain degree, deliver fluoride, which may inhibit plaque formation. They also do not shrink or require a moisture-free environment during placement.

Crown Restorations

Full coverage metal crowns are used to protect the surface of the endodontically treated tooth from further injury and to provide renewed height, shape, and function of severely deformed, fractured teeth. However, preparing the tooth to receive the crown can weaken the tooth. Porcelain-fused-to-metal (PFM) crowns are more cos-metically pleasing than metal crowns. With any type of full-coverage crown, careful evaluation of tooth size, stage of tooth development, and oral habits of the patient is imperative to achieve successful results. In many patients, installing full-coverage crowns, whether metal or porcelain-fused-to-metal, is unwise. Crown therapy is the best choice of restoration of the posterior, chewing teeth (Fig. 12-19). Creation of a metal shield around the tooth protects it from chip fractures but does not prevent "catastrophic" fracture. Crowns require a great deal of effort in terms of design and preparation; installing a crown is therefore an advanced procedure.

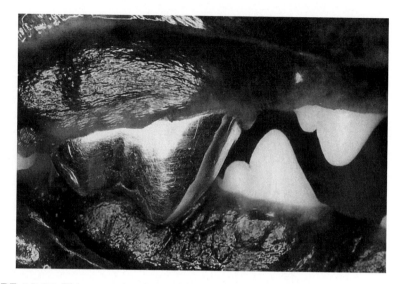

FIGURE 12-20 This crown has been placed over the right maxillary canine tooth to restore its form and function.

Metal crowns may provide renewed height, shape, and function to the tooth (Fig. 12-20). However, the clinician must be careful to avoid building the crown too high, or torque forces will accumulate. Metal crowns are custom made and require preparation of the tooth and construction of a model.

ORTHODONTICS

The term *orthodontics* refers to the correction of dental malocclusions. Before accepting the patient for orthodontic correction, the practitioner must advise the client of potential legal and ethical implications of these procedures. The client should sign a release, approved by the practitioner's attorney (Box 12-3).

Bite Evaluation

Bite evaluation entails more than just observing the incisor relationship. Although the incisor relationship is important, the complete dentition of the mouth must be evaluated. *[Dentition. Natural teeth as a unit in the dental arches.]* The classes of occlusion are Normal, Class I, Class II, Class III, and Unclassified. Normal occlusion is a scissor bite in which the lower incisors occlude on the cingulum on the palatal surface of the upper incisors. *[Cingulum. The ledge on the cervical third of the palatal surface of the crowns of the incisor teeth.]* The upper and lower premolars are in an interdigitated relationship with the maxillary teeth buccal to the mandibular teeth. The upper and lower arches are symmetric.

BOX 12-3
Sample Agreement and Consent Form*

Agreement and consent for orthodontics

The correction of malocclusions in animals has moral, ethical, and legal implications. In addition, the rules of many breed clubs and organizations state that any animal that has been altered is subject to disqualification from showing.

Because many orthodontic conditions are inherited, we strongly recommend that such animals treated for orthodontic conditions not be used for breeding purposes. Such an animal should be neutered, rendering it incapable of being shown in conformation classes.

We believe that all pets are entitled to a comfortable, functional bite. There is nothing wrong with the correction of an acquired malocclusion, but please don't ask us to be an accomplice to fraud.

My signature authorizing treatment indicates that I have read and understand the above information.

Signature of Client/Owner: _____ Date: _____

*The following release is a sample only.

Class I malocclusion

Patients with Class I malocclusion have a normal occlusion with one or more teeth out of alignment or rotated. Class I malocclusion may include any of the following characteristics: (1) a shift in the interdigitation relationship of the maxillary and mandibular premolars; (2) an anterior crossbite; (3) base narrow mandibular canine teeth; and (4) posterior crossbite.

Anterior crossbite is a common abnormal occlusion wherein one or more of the lower incisors are anterior to the upper incisors and, most important, the rest of the teeth occlude normally. A level bite is an abnormal occlusal pattern wherein the upper and lower incisors occlude cusp to cusp. This extremely punishing malocclusion results in premature wear to the incisors and the predisposition to periodontal and, to a lesser extent, endodontic disease. In base narrow or lingually displaced canine teeth the tips of the mandibular canine teeth are displaced lingually and occlude on the hard palate. Base narrow mandibular canines may also occur in Class II occlusions. Rostrally angled maxillary canine teeth can be unilateral or bilateral and are most frequently seen in Shetland sheepdogs. The maxillary canine tooth erupts at an angle, creating interference with the mandibular canine tooth; otherwise, the occlusion is normal. (This condition is also known as *lancing* or *spearing*.) Besides Shetland sheepdogs, other breeds of dogs and cats may have rostrally angled maxillary canine teeth. A posterior crossbite is an abnormal occlusion in which one or more mandibular premolars or molars occlude buccal to their occlusal counterparts.

Class II malocclusion

In Class II malocclusion the lower premolars and molars are positioned behind (distal to) the normal relationship. This malocclusion may also be termed *brachygnathism, overshot, overbite, reverse scissor bite, retrusive mandible,* and *distal mandibular excursion.*

Class III malocclusion

In Class III malocclusion the lower premolars and molars are positioned ahead of (anterior to) the normal relationship. Other terms for Class III malocclusion are *prognathism, undershot, protrusive mandible,* and *mesial mandibular excursion.*

Wry bite

A wry bite is an abnormal occlusion caused by a difference in length of the two maxillae and mandibles. This malocclusion is reported to be genetically transmitted and can result in a variety of different jaw relationships. A wry bite is characterized by asymmetry of the head caused by the failure of the midline of the maxilla to oppose the midline of the mandible.

Dental Models

Dental models are made for orthodontic evaluation and treatment and the manufacture of restorative crowns. Many instruments and materials are used (Box 12-4). The following is a fundamental technique that provides basic information on the creation of a model. All techniques require instruction and practice.

Orthodontic correction usually requires a three-stage process. In the first stage, an impression and dental model are made. An appliance is created from the model. In the second stage, the appliance is placed in the patient's mouth using orthodontic cement. Once the appliance is in place, the patient is carefully monitored at home and is returned to the practice for periodic rechecks. The third stage is the removal of the appliance after treatment is complete (Box 12-5).

Materials for making models

Impression trays may be purchased from commercial sources (Fig. 12-21). Trays designed specifically for dogs and cats should be used, although impression trays used in human dentistry will work for some veterinary impressions. Custom trays may be made out of plastic materials.

BOX 12-4
Instruments and Materials for Making Models

Impression trays
Alginate
Mixing bowls
Spatula
Dental stone
Vibrator

BOX 12-5
Orthodontics

Stage I (impression)
Radiograph materials
Impression trays
Impression material: alginate
Laboratory stone
Bite-register material
Mailing supplies for laboratory

Stage II
Orthodontic cement kit
Appliance
Orthodontic buttons
Appliance adjustment instruments
Hand scaler
Ultrasonic scaler
Flour pumice
Low-speed handpiece with new prophy cup
Power cord
Elastics

Stage III
Ultrasonic scaler
Band-removing forceps
Prophy angle, cups, and paste

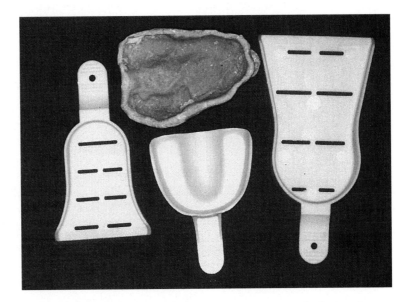

FIGURE 12-21 A variety of trays are necessary to take impressions.

When mixed with water, alginate forms an agar suspension that hardens to a gel in minutes. The actual rate of this process depends on the chemical formulation. Fast-setting and normal-setting varieties of alginate are available. Fast-setting alginate hardens in 1 to 2 minutes and is also known as *Type I alginate*. Normal-setting alginate sets in 2 to 4.5 minutes and is known as *Type II alginate*. The setting rate of alginate also varies according to water and environmental temperatures. Heat speeds up the setting rate, whereas coldness slows it down. The trays should be tested in the mouth to make sure they fit before the alginate is mixed.

Alginate is mixed in flexible rubber mixing bowls. Either metal or plastic spatulas are used for stirring. Dental stone is hardened gypsum stone. The material is mixed, allowed to set, crushed, mixed, allowed to set once more, and then crushed again several times. Its hardness and resistance to shrinkage distinguishes dental stone from plaster of Paris, which is also frequently used. A dental vibrator is used to agitate the mixed dental stone material so that bubbles emerge and escape before hardening. Also, this vibration causes the material to flow more readily.

Technique for making models

Before alginate is mixed, the trays should be tested in the mouth. Specific product directions should always be consulted beforehand. The alginate jar should first be lightly shaken to "fluff up" the material and give it a uniform volume. Alginate is measured by volume with the measuring spoon provided (Fig. 12-22). The alginate is then placed in a mixing bowl (Fig. 12-23). A measuring cup for the water is provided with the alginate (Fig. 12-24).

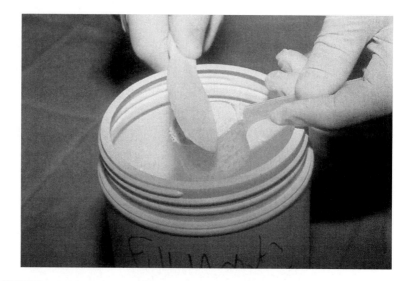

FIGURE 12-22 A dry spatula is used to level the amount in the measuring spoon.

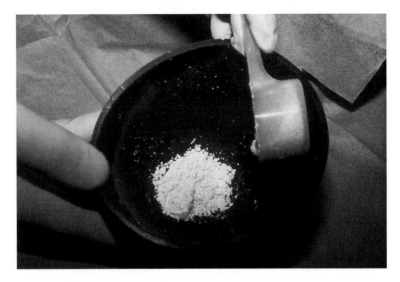

FIGURE 12-23 The alginate is placed in the rubber mixing bowl.

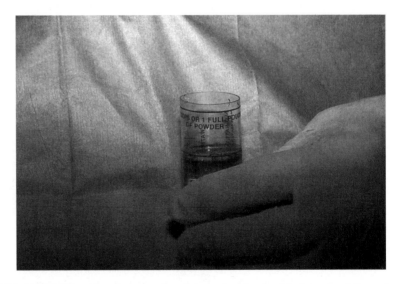

FIGURE 12-24 The directions on the alginate bottle should always be followed; usually, one scoop of alginate requires one measure of water.

FIGURE 12-25 The spatula is drawn across the bowl, mixing the alginate with the water and creating a uniform mixture.

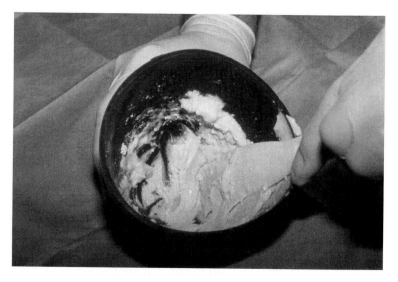

FIGURE 12-26 A spatula is used to transfer the alginate into the tray.

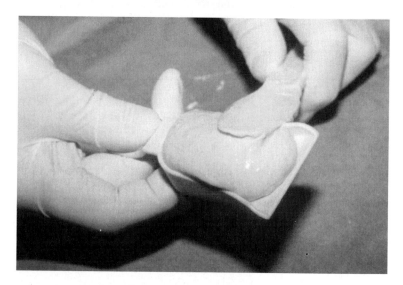

Next, the water is added to the bowl. Measuring systems are available in various sizes. The correct ratio of alginate to water is important, so the vessels should be marked if alginate from different manufacturers is being used. The alginate is mixed in a figure-eight mixing motion with a metal or plastic spatula. The bowl is rotated during mixing to ensure uniformity (Fig. 12-25). The mixed alginate is transferred by spatula to a tray of appropriate size. The alginate must be mixed, poured, and quickly placed because it will harden in only a few minutes. Once the alginate reaches a smooth consistency, it is transferred to the tray (Fig. 12-26). Spreading the material evenly in the tray with a spatula before inserting it into the mouth helps prevent the formation of air pockets and bubbles in the impression (Fig. 12-27).

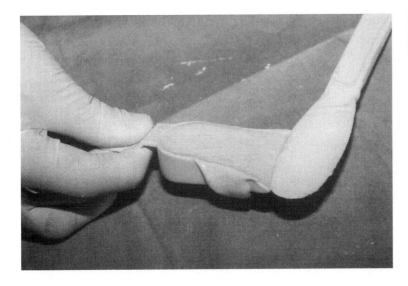

FIGURE 12-27 A spatula is used to smooth the alginate before placing it in the mouth.

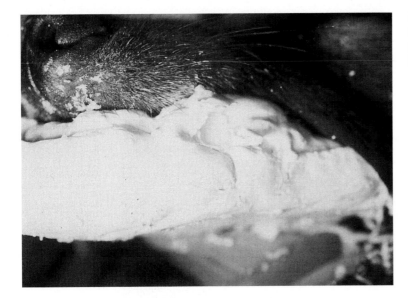

FIGURE 12-28 An alginate tray is placed in the mouth and held steady until the alginate hardens.

The tray is placed in the posterior portion of the mouth first, and the anterior portion of the tray is rotated forward and held in position until it sets (Fig. 12-28).

The last step is taking a bite registration. Two types of materials are used: bite wax and two-part bite-registration compounds. The two (maxillary and mandibular) models can be matched up with a bite registration. Bite registration material assists the lab in lining up the occlusion before laboratory work (Fig. 12-29).

Measurement of the powder and liquid is important in the mixing process. Most dental stones are measured by weight as opposed to volume (Fig. 12-30). The mea-

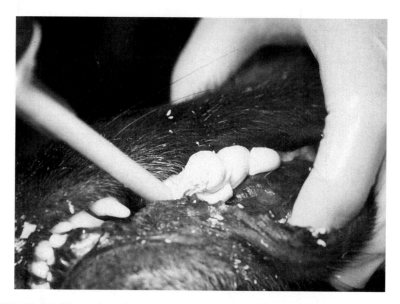

FIGURE 12-29 Bite-registration material is placed in the mouth and allowed to harden.

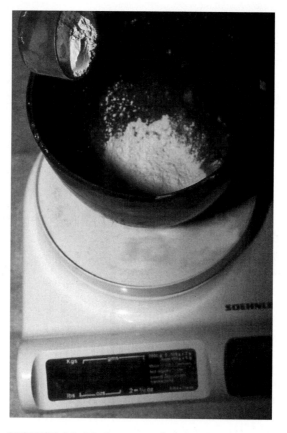

FIGURE 12-30 A gram scale is used to measure the powder portion of the dental stone.

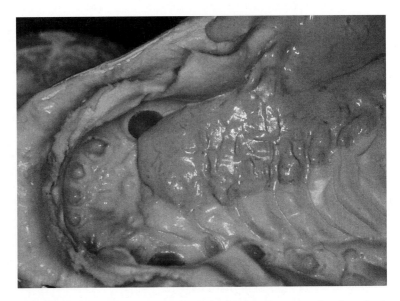

FIGURE 12-31 A dental vibrator is used to help the dental stone to flow into the impression more readily.

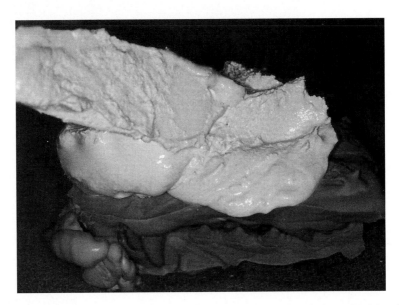

FIGURE 12-32 An inexpensive material is used to create a base for the model. After the base is placed on the model, the model is turned over to create a flat surface on the nonocclusal side.

sured water is placed in the bowl, and the dental stone is mixed. A vibrator is used to assist in the flow of the dental stone (Fig. 12-31). A base may be poured. This adds thickness to the model and may allow for easier removal of the model from the impression (Fig. 12-32).

The model should be removed from the impression as soon as it has hardened.

It is important that the alginate remain moist; if the models will not be removed immediately, the model, alginate, and tray should be kept wrapped with damp towels in a plastic bag. Removing the tray before the alginate is removed from the model may be helpful. Care should be taken not to break the teeth as the alginate is being removed (Fig. 12-33).

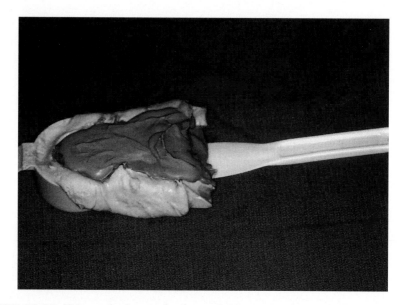

FIGURE 12-33 Using a plastic spatula, the model is separated from the impression tray by sliding the spatula between the model and tray.

Worksheet

STUDENT NAME: _____

1. Periodontal flaps are created to expose _____ and associated _____.

2. A _____ _____ and _____ _____ are used diagnostically before the procedure to determine the location of the pocket and to aid in the selection of an appropriate form of therapy.

3. The No. _____ handle is the standard scalpel handle.

4. _____ is only performed in cases where hyperplastic gingiva is present.

5. The frenoplasty procedure is designed to relieve the _____ from the gingiva.

6. _____ _____ is a general statement indicating treatment of the dental pulp.

7. Most commonly, bacteria gain entry into the pulp chamber via a _____ _____.

8. A discolored tooth, especially if pink or purple, indicates _____ _____.

9. If the tip of the crown appears _____, the patient is a candidate for a workup and evaluation of the tooth.

10. Compared with most extractions, standard root canal therapy is _____ traumatic for the patient.

11. Vital pulpotomy is indicated within _____ hours of the fracture of a mature tooth.

12. _____ _____ _____ therapy is indicated for adult teeth that are discolored and endodontically dead or that have been contaminated with long-standing infection.

13. The two most common types of files are the _____ file and the _____ file.

14. Files and reamers have two dimensions, _____ and _____.

15. _____ have blunted tips. They are used to vertically compact gutta-percha.

16. A _____ _____ is an abnormal occlusal pattern where the upper and lower incisors occlude cusp to cusp.

17. In _____ _____ or lingually displaced canine teeth the tips of the mandibular canine teeth are displaced lingually and occlude on the hard palate.

18. A _____ _____ is an abnormal occlusion caused by a difference in length of the two maxillae and mandibles.

19. _____ _____ are made for orthodontic evaluation and treatment and the manufacture of restorative crowns.

20. _____ _____ _____ are used to mix alginate. The mixing bowl is flexible, allowing better mixing.

13

Feline Dentistry

Cats have most of the conditions discussed in other chapters. However, two conditions of the oral cavity are more common in cats than they are in other species. This chapter focuses on these conditions but is not intended to minimize the importance of other diseases previously discussed with regard to all species. One condition associated with cats is lymphocytic plasmacytic stomatitis (LPS). Because severe cases often involve more than just the mucous membrane (*stomatitis* means inflammation of the mucous membrane), the term *faucitis* has been included. The fauca are located in the area where the two jaws join. The second condition discussed is feline odontoclastic resorptive lesion (FORL), which afflicts many cats and is challenging to treat.

FELINE LYMPHOCYTIC PLASMACYTIC STOMATITIS/FAUCITIS

Cause

Stomatitis is defined as an inflammation of the oral mucosa, including the buccal and labial mucosa, palate, tongue, floor of the mouth, and the gingiva. Stomatitis may be caused by local or systemic factors. Stomatitis occurs most frequently in cats and coincides with advanced periodontal disease or dental subgingival resorptive lesions, or both (Fig. 13-1).

The reason that some cats develop the painful condition called *lymphocytic plasmacytic stomatitis* (LPS) is not established. Patients with LPS have plasma cells necessary to activate immune responses. The result is the production of immunoglobulins, which play a role in immediate hypersensitivity and immune complex disease. Lymphocytes trigger cell-mediated and antibody-mediated immunity. Polymorphonuclear neutrophils, mast cells, and macrophages join in the battle. In this process the host's tissues are destroyed.

The most common form of stomatitis encountered by practitioners, feline lymphocytic plasmacytic stomatitis/faucitis is also one of the most difficult to treat successfully. Some evidence suggests that this disease is immune mediated. *[Fauces. The arch between the pharyngeal and oral cavities, formed by the tongue, tonsillar pillars, and soft palate.]* From the onset the client should be advised that initial treatment is extensive and long

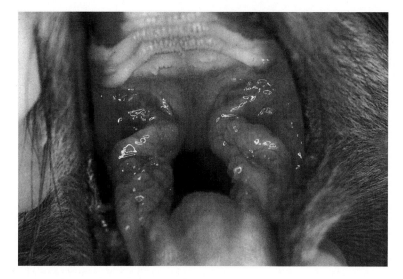

FIGURE 13-1 This patient has had severe, chronic stomatitis and faucitis for several years; the condition remains despite the extraction of all the teeth.

term, therapies have potentially dangerous side effects, and some drugs used have not been approved for use in cats. An important concept in the treatment of LPS is that treatment procedures often must be repeated.

Diagnosis

Diagnosis begins with a history and a complete physical examination of the mouth, which may require chemical restraint. The examination should include observation of the buccal mucosa, tongue, gingiva, teeth, pharynx, tonsillar region, and the hard and soft palates. All surfaces should be examined for color, shape, size, consistency, surface texture, ease of bleeding, and response to pain. Gingival bleeding is one of the earliest signs that may be noted. Inflamed gingiva and mucosa may appear swollen, cobblestone-textured, bright red, or raspberry-like, which is often symptomatic of stomatitis. Light touching of the gingiva of the patient shown in Fig. 13-2 resulted in spontaneous hemorrhage. The entire oral cavity was inflamed.

In addition to the routine complete blood count (CBC) and biochemical analysis, thyroid and autoimmune tests should be considered. For cats, FeLV and FIV tests are strongly recommended. Although these tests are often negative, they may reveal information about the cause of the individual patient's stomatitis. Most cats with classical stomatitis have elevated blood protein (hyperproteinemia) and elevated globulin (hyperglobulinemia).

One of the difficult diagnostic challenges is to determine whether the LPS is an allergic reaction to an additive in commercial pet foods. Colorants, preservatives, binders, and other chemicals are added to commercial pet foods to make them more

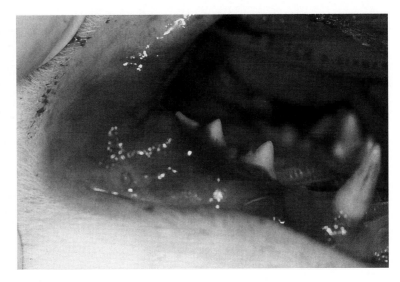

FIGURE 13-2 Gingival bleeding is one of the earliest signs observed in patients with stomatitis.

attractive to the cat and owner. If the client is cooperative, food-related causes should be investigated. Occasionally, the cause of an altered immune state is a viral infection, such as feline leukemia virus or feline immunodeficiency virus.

Biopsy is often indicated to determine probable etiology; other causes of inflammation of the oral cavity may exist. Malocclusions may cause animals to chew their cheeks, which leads to inflamed gingival and buccal tissue. Bacterial analysis of affected tissue is frustrating and seldom rewarding.

Intraoral dental radiographs are necessary for evaluation of teeth with cervical erosive disease. Radiographs are also helpful in the identification of subgingival roots if crowns are resorbed or broken off, if the apex cannot be visualized after extraction, or if the pulverization technique was used in extraction (Fig. 13-3). Hemorrhage, poor lighting, and gum tissue all can prevent full visualization of the socket. Radiographs should also be evaluated for loss of bone around the tooth. Internal (inside the root canal or pulp chamber) or external resorption of the root may be noted. The apex and periapical region of the teeth should be evaluated to determine whether endodontic disease is present.

Treatment

The first step for treatment is excellent oral hygiene. An endotracheal tube and gas anesthesia is a must to perform professional dental hygiene properly and safely.

The teeth should be cleaned and evaluated. Each tooth with indications of periodontal disease should be treated by either periodontal therapy or extraction. As with any procedure, having the proper instruments is crucial in performing a successful extraction. Oversized instruments often traumatize the patient's tissues and

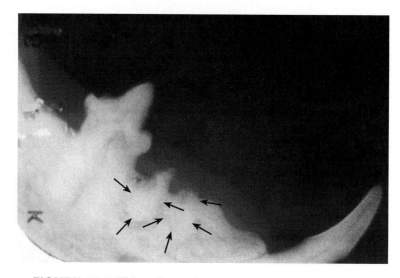

FIGURE 13-3 This radiograph shows two retained roots *(arrows)*.

can be frustrating for practitioners to use. The 301S elevator is small and well-suited to feline teeth. Root tip picks may also be beneficial. Proper lighting is essential for visualization of the root structure. Three-power magnification may help the practitioner see these small structures. A combination 3X light and binocular (not loop) glasses work well and make the work more enjoyable. The pulverization technique should be used only as a last resort. It causes excessive damage, and increases the possibility of hemorrhage. Occasionally, removal of diseased teeth and bits of root affords immediate relief. Extraction of all the premolars and molars—and occasionally all the canines and incisors as well—may be necessary. Antibiotic therapy may provide temporary relief but is usually not curative. Cortisone is usually the most effective drug for pain relief. It can be administered orally, topically, or by injection.

FELINE ODONTOCLASTIC RESORPTIVE LESION

Cause

The other condition common in cats is feline odontoclastic resorptive lesion (FORL). These lesions are also known as *neck lesions, cervical line lesions,* and *cat cavities* ("catvities"). The incidence of FORL varies according to the study, but most research suggests that a little less than one-half of the cat population is affected. The effects of FORL include resorption of the tooth and proliferation of the gingiva or pulp to cover the resulting lesion. The signs of FORL are essentially those of pain caused by the exposure of dentine. Because all patients react to pain differently, the signs may be difficult to interpret. The patient's behavior might change; some cats become aggressive or start hiding. Appetite decreases, and the animal may drop food or even hiss at it.

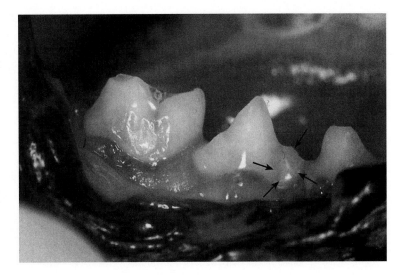

FIGURE 13-4 The left mandibular fourth premolar ($_4$P, 308) has a Grade 1 lesion on the mesial cusp.

Many theories regarding the cause of FORL have been proposed since the lesions were first reported. An early hypothesis was that they were caused by acids regurgitated with hairballs; the effect on the teeth was compared with that of humans suffering from bulimia. However, in humans the lesions tend to be on lingual surfaces, whereas in cats they occur on either side. Some researchers have suggested that the acids produced by bacteria associated with periodontal disease are responsible. However, studies have shown that periodontal disease usually follows FORL. Current research indicates that FORL may be caused by nutritional problems aggravated by unknown genetic factors.

Diagnosis

The clinical sign of inflamed gums may initially lead the clinician to suspect that FORLs are present. Some lesions are immediately apparent, and others are covered by hyperplastic gingiva. In most cases the extent of the lesion is impossible to determine by visual clinical examination alone. Dental radiographs are necessary to accurately diagnose and treat FORL.

Treatment

Lesions are classified to assist in treatment planning. Grade 1 lesions involve the enamel only and may be filled with a glass ionomer or light cure composite (Fig. 13-4). Home care may help in the prevention of future occurrences. Grade 2 lesions have invaded the dentine but have not entered the pulp. Grade 2 lesions may be filled with a glass ionomer or light cure composite (Fig. 13-5). However, the practitioner should inform the client that these lesions may persist and the restoration may not succeed. Grade 3 lesions show pulp involvement, but the crown remains intact (Fig. 13-6). In most cases,

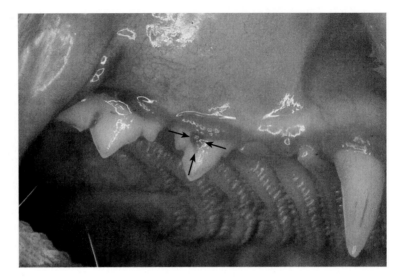

FIGURE 13-5 This Grade 2 lesion of the right maxillary third premolar (P^3, 107) has been covered by hyperplastic gingiva.

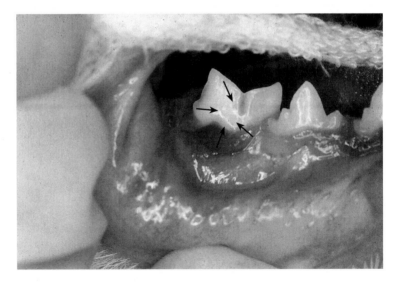

FIGURE 13-6 Grade 3 lesion of the distal root of the right mandibular first molar (M_1, 409) *(arrows)*.

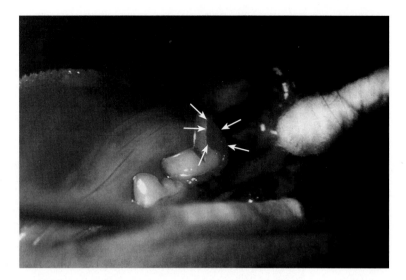

FIGURE 13-7 T Grade 4 lesion of the left mandibular first molar ($_1$M, 309) *(arrows)*.

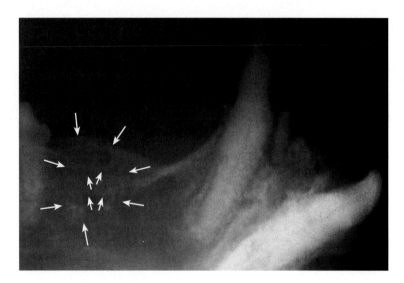

FIGURE 13-8 Resorption of the right mandibular third premolar (P$_3$, 407) *(arrows)*.

extraction is the best choice in treatment. However, some teeth may be saved by endodontic therapy followed by restoration. Grade 4 lesions show pulp involvement and resorption of the dentine surrounding the pulp (Fig. 13-7). Crown loss is evident. Extraction of the tooth is the best option. Grade 5 lesions show complete crown loss. This is the end stage of the process. If continued disease is evident after crown loss, root extraction is the best alternative. The patient in Fig. 13-8 shows advanced resorption of the crown; only remnants of the right mandibular third premolar can be visualized. Treatment in this case is not necessary.

Patients may have teeth at various stages of resorption. Generally, if one lesion is noted clinically, other lesions can be found radiographically. In some cases, treatment may be necessary, but extraction is usually the best treatment (Fig. 13-9).

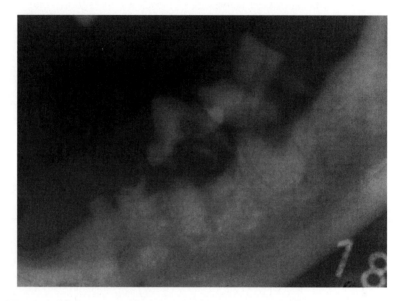

FIGURE 13-9 All these mandibular premolar and molar teeth have advanced resorptive lesions. The best treatment is extraction.

Worksheet

1. Two conditions of the oral cavity more common in cats than they are in other species are _____ _____ _____ _____ and _____ _____ _____.

2. _____ is defined as an inflammation of the oral mucosa, including the buccal and labial mucosa, palate, tongue, floor of the mouth, and gingiva.

3. _____ cells activate immune responses.

4. Altered immune state may be caused by _____ or _____.

5. In the treatment of LPS/F, each tooth with indications of periodontal disease should be treated either by periodontal therapy or _____.

6. About _____ % of the domestic cat population has FORL.

7. The lesions of FORL cause _____ of the tooth.

8. Grade _____ lesions involve the enamel only.

9. The most common treatment for FORL is _____.

10. _____ _____ are necessary to accurately diagnose and treat FORL.

14

Pocket Pet Dentistry

ROBERT B. WIGGS

This chapter discusses equipment, supplies, and techniques necessary for the basic oral examination and treatment of many rodents and lagomorphs that clients may keep as pets. Relevant anatomy is also reviewed.

GENERAL INFORMATION

Rodents

The name rodents comes from the word *rodere,* meaning "to gnaw." The rodentia order is the largest order of the mammal classification and contains a great diversity of species. Some of the smaller animals within this order that are sometimes kept as pets are the rat, mouse, guinea pig, hamster, gerbil, chinchilla, gopher, squirrel, and prairie dog.

Lagomorphs

The lagomorph order includes the domestic rabbit, hare, and cottontail. Lagomorphs were once grouped with rodents; a separate order was later created because of their distinct dental differences in the number of incisor teeth. The rabbit is the only member of this order commonly kept as a family pet.

DENTAL ANATOMY

Type of Dentition in the Rodent and Lagomorph

Most rodents and all lagomorphs are herbivores, eating leaves, grass, and other lush green plants; however, some of the rat species are omnivores that also eat certain types of meat. All species have a dental formula that features variation in tooth size and shape among the incisors, premolars, and molars. This is known as a *heterodont* form of dentition. Lagomorphs also do not have canine teeth but instead have a long diastema or edentulous (toothless) area between the incisors and cheek teeth. Animals within these groups may have deciduous and permanent teeth (diphyodont) or only permanents (monophyodonts). Although they have both upper and lower incisors, lagomorphs differ from rodents in having two rows of incisor teeth in the maxillary or upper arcade. This first row of incisors consists of two larger functional teeth; a second row of two small, rudimentary pegs, which have no known function, exists immediately behind the first row.

Type of teeth in the lagomorph

A tooth that grows continuously throughout life is known as an *aradicular hypsodont tooth*. This is the only type of tooth found in lagomorphs. Although these teeth have a clinical crown and root, they do not have a true root structure but merely additional crown that is submerged below the gumline, waiting to erupt as the tooth undergoes normal attrition or wear from mastication. This form of tooth is found in both the incisors and cheek teeth.

Type of teeth in the rodent

Two basic types of teeth are found in the rodent: the aradicular hypsodont (continuously growing tooth) and, in some species, brachyodont cheek teeth. The brachyodont tooth is the same basic tooth type found in humans: a tooth with a true crown and root that does not truly grow in size or shape once erupted. For example, guinea pigs and chinchillas have aradicular hypsodont teeth for both the incisors and cheek teeth, whereas mice and rats have hypsodont incisors and brachyodont cheek teeth (premolars and molars).

Incisor teeth of the rodent and lagomorph

The upper and lower incisor teeth of rodents and lagomorphs, not including the rudimentary incisor peg teeth of the lagomorphs, come to a chisel-type point that angles back toward the tongue. These teeth have enamel on the front and lateral sides but typically just cementum and dentine on the side toward the tongue. The cementum and dentine wear much faster than enamel, resulting in a chisel edge that is longer labially. In addition, the enamel in most of these species commonly takes on a yellow-orange tint, giving these teeth their typical bright yellow appearance. These teeth curve through the jaws during development, resulting in their long curved shape or form. The location of the apex of these teeth varies with the species of animal. In most species the apex of the maxillary incisor teeth lies beneath the edentulous diastema. However, in rats and mice, the mandibular incisor apex is distal to the roots of the last cheek tooth, whereas rabbits and chinchillas usually have their apex near the mesial surface of the first cheek tooth.

Hypsodont cheek teeth of the rodent and lagomorph

Because of their unique function, hypsodont cheek teeth usually have an angled rather than flat occlusal table. In some species, such as the guinea pig, the cheek teeth angle to an actual chisel point somewhat similar to that of the incisors. However, other species, such as the rabbit, only have a very slight angulation to the occlusal bed. The chisel-point tip of the maxillary teeth is buccal or toward the face, angling up toward the soft tissue of the hard palate. The bevel of the mandibular cheek teeth goes in the opposite direction. The chisel point is on the lingual side, and the tooth's occlusal table angles down toward the soft tissue of the cheek. These wear patterns are due to the fact that the maxillary cheek teeth are spread wider apart from the midline than are the mandibular teeth. This is known as an *ansiognathic,* or naturally unequal, jaw relationship, in which the upper dental arch is slightly larger than the lower.

Periodontal Ligament

The periodontal ligament (PDL) of the aradicular hypsodont teeth differs from that of adult brachyodont teeth because of the presence of an intermediate plexus through the center of the PDL between its tooth attachment and its bone attachment. This plexus allows for continuously growing teeth to move upward as they grow. Otherwise, the periodontal ligament would hold firmly to the tooth and prevent its continued eruption.

Adult Rodent Dental Formula

The adult rodent dental formula is as follows:

Hamster:

$$2 \times (I\ 1/1,\ C\ 0/0,\ P\ 0/0,\ M\ 2\text{-}3/2\text{-}3) = 12\ \text{to}\ 16\ \text{total teeth}$$

Rat:

$$2 \times (I\ 1/1,\ C\ 0/0,\ P\ 0/0,\ M\ 2\text{-}3/2\text{-}3) = 12\ \text{to}\ 16\ \text{total teeth}$$

Gerbil:

$$2 \times (I\ 1/1,\ C\ 0/0,\ P\ 0/0,\ M\ 3/3) = 16\ \text{total teeth}$$

Guinea pig and chinchilla:

$$2 \times (I\ 1/1,\ C\ 0/0,\ P\ 1/1,\ M\ 3/3) = 20\ \text{total teeth}$$

Squirrel:

$$2 \times (I\ 1/1,\ C\ 0/0,\ P\ 1\text{-}2/1,\ M\ 3/3) = 20\ \text{to}\ 22\ \text{total teeth}$$

Adult Lagomorph Dental Formula

The adult lagomorph dental formula is as follows:

Rabbit:

$$2 \times (I\ 2/1,\ C\ 0/0,\ P\ 3/2,\ M\ 2\text{-}3/3) = 26\ \text{to}\ 28\ \text{total teeth}$$

Hare:

$$2 \times (I\ 2/1,\ C\ 0/0,\ P\ 3/2,\ M\ 3/3) = 28\ \text{total teeth}$$

INSTRUMENTS AND EQUIPMENT USED TO TREAT RODENTS AND LAGOMORPHS

The following instruments and equipment are used in the treatment of oral disorders in rodents and lagomorphs:

Towels can be used for restraint by gently wrapping the patient in them or for patient comfort by providing a warm, soft bed during the procedure.

An **anesthesia chamber** is a clear Plexiglas compartment used with an inhalant anesthetic for initial sedation before masking or intubation.

Anesthesia masks can be used for induction of anesthesia before intubation or for the maintenance of anesthesia using an off-and-on mask approach during the actual dental procedure.

Anesthesia machines may also be used if preferred by the clinician.

Anesthesia is available in two forms: injectable and inhalant. Injectables or combination injectables such as ketamine, acepromazine, and others usually result in a longer recovery time than inhalants. Inhalants, in the form of volatilized liquids such as isoflurane, are preferred for most procedures.

A **laryngoscope with a small pediatric straight blade** is used for endotracheal intubation to maintain the airway and administer anesthesia.

An **otoscope with ear cones** is used for oral examination of small mouths to visualize the teeth and oral cavity. In addition, it can be used as an aid in passing endotracheal tubes or IV catheters used as endotracheal tubes.

Endotracheal tubes in sizes 1.5, 2.0, 2.5, or 3.0 Cole or a standard endotracheal tube may be used depending on the patient's size. A wire guide in the tubes makes passage much easier (Fig. 14-1).

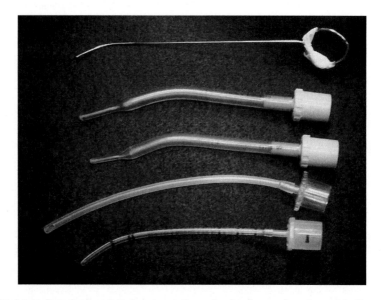

FIGURE 14-1 Standard and Cole-type endotracheal tubes and a wire guide for use in the tubes during placement.

IV catheters (12-14 gauge) can be used as an endotracheal tube for smaller rodents if the stylet is removed. These catheters can often be passed with the use of an otoscope and ear cone as a laryngoscope.

Umbilical tape is used to anchor the endotracheal tube by snugly tying it to the tube and then behind the pet's head.

Swabs are used during dental procedures to clear the oral cavity of saliva, moisture, and debris.

Explorers/probes are used to examine teeth and their associated structures.

Handpieces, both high-speed and low-speed, can be used with burs to shape, trim, prepare, or resect teeth.

Cheek retractors are single-bladed instruments that retract the cheek on a single side or double-bladed instruments with a spring wire that spread both buccal folds at the same time (Fig. 14-2).

Tongue retractors are generally instruments with a single, flat blade used to move the tongue away from the area to be inspected or treated (Fig. 14-3).

Mouth gags aid in keeping the mouth open during inspection and treatment. Most are spring activated, although some are mechanical (Fig. 14-4).

Burs are used for most treatments. The three most common types are the carbide round ball, carbide crosscuts, and white stone points. Of the carbide burs, the 699L tapered crosscut and #1 and #2 round ball burs have been found helpful in many cases. Of the white stone abrasive points, the flame shape is a good selection.

Floats (rabbit float, bone files/rasps, diamond burs, carbide burs, white stones) are instruments used to level an uneven occlusive table of the teeth. Many instruments can be used for this purpose. The burs and abrasive points can be used easily and quickly on the incisors but can be difficult to use safely and carefully on

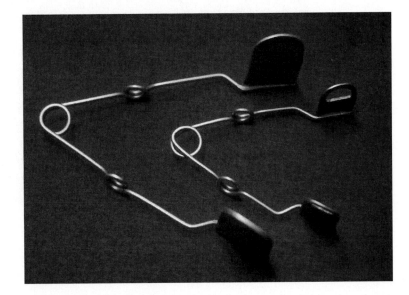

FIGURE 14-2 Spring cheek retractors used to move the abundant cheek pouch tissue away for improved visualization of the teeth.

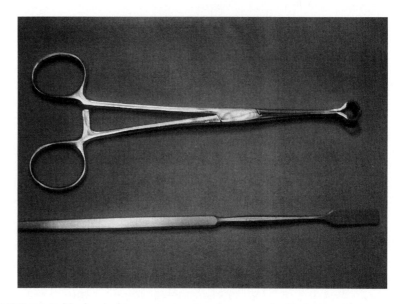

FIGURE 14-3 Mechanical tongue-retracting forceps and a blade-type tongue retractor.

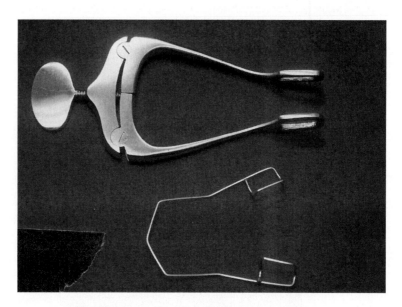

FIGURE 14-4 Mechanical and spring mouth gags.

the cheek teeth because of the bulky size of the handpieces and poor accessibility. The hand floats used in the small mouths of rodents and lagomorphs are typically either modified bone files or rasps. The rasps cut both on the push and pull stroke, whereas the files typically cut only on the pull stroke. The author prefers files that cut on the pull stroke. The BF4 bone rasp (Cislak, Inc., Glenview, IL 60025) and the Howard 12 bone file (Schein, Inc., Port Washington, NY 11050) are two of the instruments that can be used for floating many cheek teeth (Fig. 14-5).

The **rabbit molar rasp** is a float specifically developed for use in rabbits. Most have a large handle for better control and a working end that is similar to a bone rasp. Although listed as a rabbit molar rasp, the J-51RR (Jorgensen Labs, Inc., Loveland, CO 80538) is actually a file; it is one of the better known instruments of this group.

Molar or cheek teeth cutters are frequently modified hard-tissue nippers, pin and wire cutting pliers, or sided cutting rongeurs. However, some have been developed specifically for use in rabbits (Fig. 14-6).

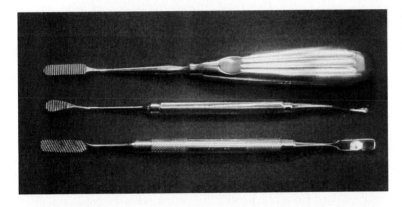

FIGURE 14-5 Rasps and files used for floating of teeth in rodents and lagomorphs.

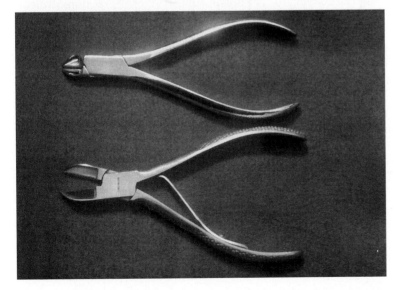

FIGURE 14-6 Molar or cheek teeth cutters used for removing small tooth spurs.

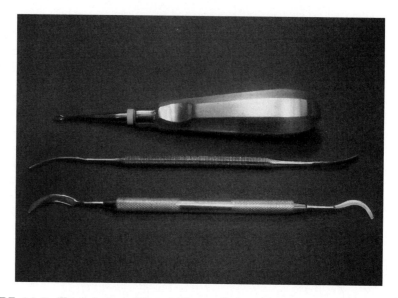

FIGURE 14-7 *(Top to bottom):* Winged Elevator® (Dentalaire, Inc., Fountain Valley, CA 92708), double-ended rabbit/rodent elevator, and a Crossley Rabbit Luxator® (Jorgensen Labs, Inc., Loveland, CO 80538).

Elevators are used to work circumferentially around the tooth down into the periodontal ligament space to aid in the tooth's removal. Blunted injection needles, sizes 25- to 18-gauge, can often be used for this function in rodents and lagomorphs. However, standard elevators can also be used, such as the No.1 and No. 2 Winged Elevators® (Dentalaire, Inc., Fountain Valley, CA 92708), 301 apical elevators, and Crossley Rabbit Luxators (Jorgensen Labs, Inc., Loveland, CO 80538) (Fig. 14-7).

Extraction forceps are used to grasp teeth loosened by elevation or disease. Most incisors can be handled with small animal extraction forceps. For the cheek teeth a small 90-degree angled Halstead Mosquito forceps or an angled root tip forceps can be useful. Some extraction forceps are specifically designed for use in rabbits (Fig. 14-8).

Bone replacement materials are used to pack into areas where abscess or dental disease has resulted in bone loss. Two of the more commonly used are Consil® (Nutramax Labs, Baltimore, MD 21236) and HTR® (Bioplant, Inc., South Norwalk, CT 06854). These may be combined with an antibiotic or other medicament when placed in a bony void.

Paper points are commonly employed to apply medicaments to exposed pulps.

Calcium hydroxide is commonly used in either a powder or paste form. It is placed over the exposed pulp of a tooth in an attempt to maintain its vitality.

Restorative is ordinarily either a temporary filling material such as Cavit® or one of the glass ionomer restorative materials.

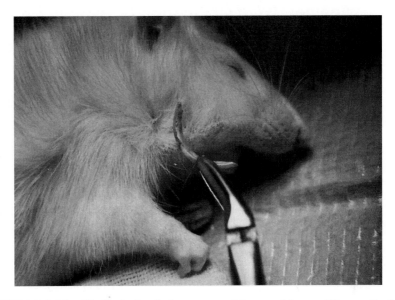

FIGURE 14-8 Mandibular incisor being extracted from a white rat. Observe the length of the tooth and its clinical root in relation to the length of the patient's jaw. This demonstrates that even teeth that are long in relation to the associated jaw can be safely extracted with proper equipment and technique.

COMMON ORAL PROBLEMS AND DISEASES

Common problems in rodents and lagomorphs are gingivitis, periodontal disease, enamel hypocalcification, tooth caries, fractured teeth, malocclusion, tongue-tied syndrome, tooth overgrowth, abscessed teeth, cheek pouch impaction, stomatitis, oral tumors, and slobbers.

Gingivitis

Typically, gingivitis in the front of the mouth in rodents and lagomorphs is due to trauma to the mouth caused by rough edges on watering devices and food bowls. Treatment includes removal, repair, or replacement of the defective device causing the trauma. Once the source of irritation is removed, most patients respond positively without further treatment. However, if the situation warrants, the area or lesion can be treated with multiple coats of tincture of myrrh and benzoin or antibiotic ointments. Antibiotics may also be administered by injection or added to food or drinking water.

Periodontal Disease

Periodontal disease is generally found only in the cheek teeth of rodents with brachyodont teeth, such as mice and rats. Treatment consists of routine cleaning of the teeth and, if warranted, extractions and administration of antibiotics.

Enamel Hypocalcification or Hypoplasia

Undermineralized areas of enamel may be seen occasionally on incisor teeth. This may appear as a chalky white or brown discoloration on the facial side of the tooth. Enamel hypocalcification or hypoplasia generally results from either a nutritional imbalance or an infection or inflammation that temporarily depresses enamel production. Generally the only treatment required is correction of the initiating cause. The teeth seldom require any direct treatment, unless the weakened area of the tooth results in a tooth fracture.

Tooth Caries

True caries are generally found in only the cheek teeth of rodents with brachyodont teeth. Caries are considered uncommon, but this may be because cheek teeth are difficult for most practitioners to routinely examine. The caries may be on the crown surface, but many are found on the root surfaces, making them even more difficult to detect. Treatment is generally extraction, although fillings with glass ionomers have been used in some cases in an attempt to maintain the teeth as vital and functional.

Malocclusion

Malocclusions can be classified in two basic categories: traumatic and atraumatic.

Traumatic malocclusions

Traumatic injuries to the teeth can result in broken crowns, which may cause overgrowth of the opposing tooth because of the lack of normal attrition or wear.
1. Treatment of the overgrowth of the opposing tooth can generally be controlled by the periodic floating or odontoplasty of the tooth in question.
2. Treatment of the fractured tooth includes initial inspection to determine whether the tooth's pulp has been exposed. If it has but the tooth is still vital, a pulp capping should be performed to improve the chances of maintaining the tooth's vitality. If the tooth is nonvital, it and its opposing tooth may eventually require extraction.

Atraumatic malocclusions

Atraumatic malocclusions are normally not attributed to trauma; hence the name. Ordinarily, atraumatic malocclusions are caused by genetic or hereditary factors and nutritional and other physiologic changes in teeth, joints, symphysis, or bone that result in improper tooth alignment. Atraumatic malocclusion is found in three basic forms:
1. Short maxillary diastema results in the maxillary incisor teeth being too far lingual in their eruption and therefore failing to meet properly with the mandibular incisors. This results in the overgrowth of one or more of the incisor teeth. This condition typically manifests within the first year of the animal's life. Treatment entails control of the overgrowth by routine floating of the incisor teeth.
2. Mandibular drift is thought to result when certain changes, stimulated by genetics, nutrition, or other physiologic action, occur in the mandible itself, the temporomandibular joint, or the mandibular symphysis. These changes allow for drift of the mandible or teeth, resulting in a malocclusion of the incisors or

the cheek teeth (premolars and molars). This condition usually makes itself known after 2 years of age and has a poor long-term prognosis because of secondary complications; the client should be notified of this fact. Treatment includes the routine floating of the affected cheek and incisors and symptomatic treatment of other secondary conditions that may arise. This may include the use of antibiotics, antiinflammatories, and fluids.

3. Improper wear is a result of chewing and eating behavior. Treatment consists of dietary correction, if required, and the periodic floating of any tooth overgrowth.

Tongue-Tied Condition

The tongue-tied condition occurs when the mandibular cheek teeth grow until they reach the inside of the maxillary cheek teeth and then grow across the top of the tongue, pinning the tongue to the roof of the mouth. Treatment involves cutting of the overgrown teeth to release the tongue and possible routine floating of these teeth in the future to prevent recurrence. In addition, antibiotics, antiinflammatories, fluids, hand feeding, and other supportive therapies may be required during the healing stages. Once this condition occurs, the long term prognosis may be poor.

Incisor Tooth Overgrowth

When not complicated by cheek tooth involvement, incisor tooth overgrowth (Fig. 14-9) can usually be treated and controlled by one of the two following methods:

1. Odontoplasty (floating or reconfiguration), which reestablishes a functional occlusion.

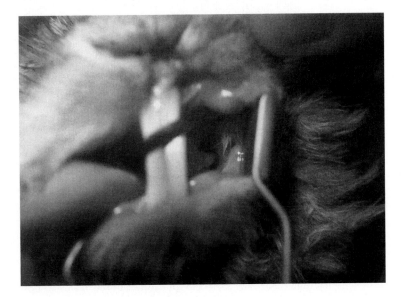

FIGURE 14-9 Improper incisor growth in a rabbit. Note the angular appearance of the maxillary and mandibular incisor occlusion.

2. Extraction, which removes the occlusal interference and trauma while establishing a functional occlusion.

Molar Tooth Overgrowth

Once molar tooth overgrowth (Fig. 14-10) and root inflammation begin, a serious, life-threatening disease process usually eventually ensues. Molar tooth overgrowth results in a chronic inflammatory disease that causes gradual weight loss and many secondary health problems. The condition can be controlled by odontoplasty, antibiotics, antiinflammatories, and supportive therapies.

Abscessed Tooth

Diseased teeth may develop endodontic or periodontic abscesses. Treatment may involve endodontic procedures, but extraction of the diseased tooth is generally best. The actual abscess may require incision, drainage, and treatment.

Cheek Pouch Impaction

Occasionally, food becomes impacted in the cheek pouches, causing mild buccal irritation or stomatitis. Treatment consists of removal of the impacted material and treatment of the stomatitis with an antibiotic ointment.

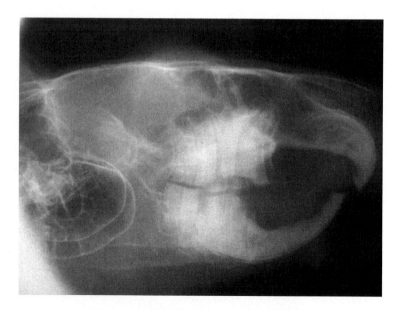

FIGURE 14-10 Lateral extra oral radiograph of a chinchilla's cheek teeth using a No. 4 dental film. Notice the irregular appearance of the occlusion of the cheek teeth.

Stomatitis

Most cases of stomatitis are secondary to another cause, such as food impaction, discussed previously, or hypovitaminosis C, which results in scurvy. Scurvy leads to gingivitis, periodontal disease, oral hemorrhage, mobile or lost teeth, anorexia, and loss of body weight. Treatment should be immediately initiated with vitamin C supplements and supportive therapy, which may include fluid therapy and tube feeding. The diet should be enhanced with fruits and vegetables rich in vitamin C. If a commercial diet is being used, its expiration date should be closely inspected because the vitamin C in commercial diets gradually depletes with time. For this reason, these diets are usually dated for safety.

Oral Tumors

Many oral tumors can be found in rodents and lagomorphs. Treatment is generally either incisional or excisional biopsy and treatment in accordance with histologic findings.

Slobbers

Slobbers, or wet dewlap, is a condition in which excess salivation results in a moist dermatitis. Many of the previously described oral diseases may cause this condition. Treatment must include control of the initiating disease, but the dermatitis is treated by clipping of the fur or hair, cleansing, and treatment of the area with topical antibiotics.

PREPARATION FOR PROCEDURES

Preanesthesia Examination

The preanesthesia examination has two parts. The first is a thorough general examination in preparation for anesthesia. The second is a brief survey of the oral cavity to obtain an idea of the type of problems that may be encountered so that appropriate equipment, instruments, and supplies can be prepared. However, the initial oral survey may not be particularly informative because of the small size of the oral cavity and anatomy in these small pets. The use of an otoscope with an ear cone inserted into the mouth sometimes allows a degree of visualization of the teeth and oral cavity in tolerant pets (Fig. 14-11).

Preanethesia Preparation

Preanesthesia preparations are an integral part of the procedure. The planned procedure and its risks should be discussed with the client. Additionally, an estimate of cost and procedure time should be provided so that clients do not become unnecessarily anxious during the procedure. If the client will not be present during the

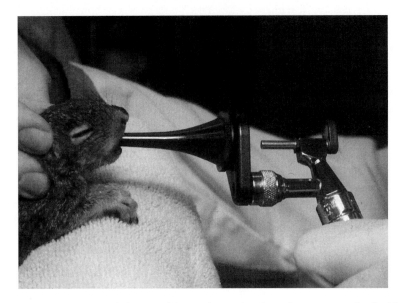

FIGURE 14-11 Otoscope being used for oral examination of a young squirrel with a traumatic tooth injury.

procedure, a contingency plan should be arranged in case any additional problems arise or are discovered during the procedure. If the client has failed to provide direction or cannot be contacted during a procedure, only the agreed-upon procedures and those necessary to maintain the patient should be performed. Preoperative antibiotics can, if indicated, be given before anesthesia as well as other indicated preoperative agents. Preanesthesia restriction of food and water is often not required in rodents or lagomorphs because their digestive system does not ordinarily allow for ingesta regurgitation. In compromised patients, even short-term nutritional restriction may be contraindicated. There are many different anesthetic agents, many of which are injectables (Table 14-1).

Inhalant Anesthesia

Ether has been used in the past as an inhalant anesthetic, but because of its flammability and other problems, it should probably not be used in a general practice setting. Halothane works well in most cases, but isoflurane is without a doubt currently the inhalant anesthetic of choice for general usage in rodents and lagomorphs.

Anesthesia Induction

Induction of anesthesia is ordinarily done in one of three ways: (1) restraint and use of injectables; (2) restraint and masking with an inhalant form of anesthesia; or (3) placement of the pet in an anesthesia chamber and use of an inhalant anesthetic.

TABLE 14-1 Injectable Anesthesia and Sedation

				SPECIES		
	Rabbit	Guinea pig	Chinchilla	Hamster	Gerbil	Rat
Ketamine injectable	20-50 mg/kg IM	20-60 mg/kg IM/IP	20-60 mg/kg IM/IP	40-200 mg/kg IP	40-100 mg/kg IP	40-100 mg/kg IM/IP
Ketamine and acepromazine injectable	25-40 mg/kg + 0.25-1.0 mg/kg; IM	20-50 mg/kg + 0.5-1.0 mg/kg; IM	20-40 mg/kg + 0.5 mg/kg; IM	50-150 mg/kg + 2.5-5.0 mg/kg; IM	DO NOT USE; NOT RECOMMENDED	50-150 mg/kg + 2.5-5.0 mg/kg; IM
Ketamine and diazepam injectable	20-40 mg/kg + 5-10 mg/kg; IM	20-50 mg/kg + 3-5 mg/kg; IM	20-40 mg/kg + 3-5 mg/kg; IM	40-150 mg/kg + 5 mg/kg; IM	40-150 mg/kg + 3-5 mg/kg; IM	40-100 mg/kg + 3-5 mg/kg; IM
Ketamine and xylazine injectable	20-40 mg/kg + 3-5 mg/kg; IM	20-44 mg/kg + 3-5 mg/kg; IM	35 mg/kg + 5 mg/kg; IM	50-150 mg/kg + 5-10 mg/kg; IM	50-70 mg/kg + 2-3 mg/kg; IM	90 mg/kg + 5 mg/kg; IM

IP, Intraperitoneal; *IM*, intramuscular; *IV*, intravenous.

Anesthesia Maintenance

Maintenance of anesthesia is also typically accomplished in one of three ways: injection, alternating off/on masking, or intubation. The use of injectables has many more cons than pros. Drawbacks include injection site abscesses, hair loss at the site of injection, a more prolonged recovery time, and greater sensitivity in chronically ill animals. The only positive feature is that injectable anesthesia can be performed on almost any animal fairly easily. Once an animal is induced, the technique of alternating off/on masking allows time for treatment of minor oral conditions and easily reached incisor teeth (Fig. 14-12). This technique can also be used for cheek teeth and other more complicated treatments in the mouth, but it can greatly prolong the time needed to accomplish the treatment. Animals maintained in this fashion generally recover fairly rapidly.

When intubation is accomplished, treatment in the oral cavity, especially the cheek teeth, is easier to perform and recovery is usually quick and uneventful.

Intubation

Intubation of rodents and lagomorphs can be difficult and frustrating. However, with routine practice, intubation can be accomplished in many of these small pets. The following are six major methods for intubation:

Blind intubation

Used primarily in rabbits, chinchillas, and larger rodents and lagomorphs, blind intubation is often the most simple and effective way of intubating these animals. An

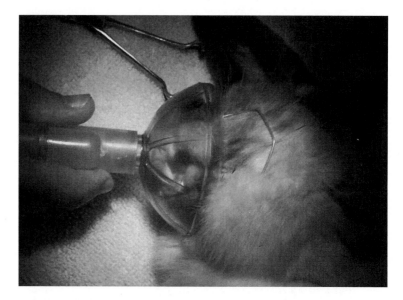

FIGURE 14-12 Rabbit being masked for a dental procedure using isoflurane as the anesthesia agent.

endotracheal tube (size 2.0, 2.5, 3.0) is cut to the appropriate length depending on the animal to be intubated. A wire guide is made with a loop on one end for easy extraction from the connector end of the tube. The wire is cut so that it is approximately 1 mm short of the end of the tube. This reduces the chance of trauma to the soft tissues caused by the wire sticking out of the tube. The wire is bent 1 cm back from the insertion end at a gentle 45-degree angle. A section of umbilical tape is tied around the tube for its eventual anchorage. The tube is then inserted into the oral cavity with the bent tip angled toward the tongue. The bend in the wire should make contact with the roof of the mouth, forcing the tip downward into the trachea. Typically, a light gagging reflex will be induced, and with transparent tubes the fluxing of moisture is visible with each breath. The umbilical tape should then be tied behind the ears to anchor and stabilize the tube. Should the first attempt fail, another attempt should be made before attempting the next intubation technique.

Pediatric laryngoscope

Used primarily in rabbits, chinchillas, and larger rodents and lagomorphs, pediatric laryngoscopes with pediatric blades can sometimes lead to easy intubation. Although the angled pediatric blade can be used, the straight blade seems to more accurately provide the needed visualization for intubation. The lighted blade is first inserted into the mouth. The endotracheal tube with a wire stylet is then introduced parallel to and outside of the blade track to maximize visualization of intubation. The endotracheal tube should then be secured by tying umbilical tape around the tube and behind the ears. An alternative procedure, which is sometimes easier, is to first pass a No. 5 French urinary catheter into the trachea. Then the endotracheal tube is slid down over the urinary catheter, and finally the urinary catheter is removed. The endotracheal tube should then be secured by tying umbilical tape around the tube and behind the ears.

Otoscope with endotracheal tube or IV catheter

Intubation using an otoscope with an endotracheal tube or IV catheter is primarily used with rats, hamsters, gerbils, chinchillas, and smaller rodents and lagomorphs. This form of intubation calls for the use of an ear cone in a size appropriate for the size and depth of the animal's oral cavity. The otoscope is advanced until the laryngeal area can be identified. An endotracheal tube can be advanced beside the otoscope and then into the trachea by visual placement. The plastic sheath of an IV catheter with the stylet removed can be advanced down the actual inside of the otoscope into the trachea. The otoscope and cone must then be removed without disturbing the positioning of the catheter. The catheter or endotracheal tube must then be anchored by umbilical tape, which is tied to the catheter and then around the animal's head. The use of IV catheters for intubation allows for a patent airway, but regulation of a gas anesthesia through such small devices can sometimes be trying. Additionally, any small endotracheal tube, especially the diminutive IV catheters used as endotracheal tubes, can quickly become blocked by mucus or debris. Therefore their patency should be closely observed and maintained.

Fiberoptic endoscope

Fiberoptic endoscopes are used in all sizes of rodents and lagomorphs. With the use of a fiberoptic endoscope, the laryngeal area can usually be located for passing an endotracheal tube by visual confirmation.

Retro guide

Retro guide intubation can be used in all sizes of rodents and lagomorphs. However, this method can be traumatic and highly irritating to the trachea and should be used only when the two previously described techniques have failed. In this technique a needle is inserted through the midventral neck region between two of the tracheal rings and directed toward the head. The needle should be stopped as soon as it penetrates the trachea. A monofilament suture is then passed through the needle into the trachea and gently pushed until it exits into the mouth. The end of the suture is then grasped and passed through the endotracheal tube. The tube is then slid down over the suture into the trachea. Both ends of the suture should be held firmly to provide a smooth, taut guideline for the tube. Once the tube is in the trachea, the suture and needle are removed from the neck and the endotracheal tube adjusted to the appropriate depth. The endotracheal tube should then be secured by tying umbilical tape around the tube and behind the ears.

Tracheotomy intubation

Tracheotomy intubations may be performed in all sizes of rodents and lagomorphs. However, this method should be reserved only for special or critical cases in which intubation is absolutely required and more conservative techniques have failed. In this technique a tracheotomy is performed by making a longitudinal incision over the trachea midway between the larynx and thoracic inlet. Proper clipping of the hair and disinfection of the site with surgical scrub solutions should be performed. A stab incision is then made between two of the tracheal rings, and the endotracheal tube is passed into the trachea and then anchored with umbilical tape, which is tied to the tube and then around the animal's neck to prevent accidental extubation.

Stabilization and Monitors

After intubation, the patient should be monitored for stability and safety. A spare tube should be kept close at hand for emergencies. In most cases a 500-ml bag and pediatric set of anesthesia tubes can be used. Oxygen flow should be at a minimum of 500 ml, and the isoflurane set at approximately 1% to 2.5% for maintenance. Once every 2 minutes, the tube patency should be checked by light positive pressure ventilation. If moisture or mucus blocks the tube, the tube should be disconnected and an open-end tom cat catheter inserted down the tube. A syringe can be attached and light negative pressure used to remove the debris. Should patency not be immediately reestablished, the tube should be removed and the patient masked until the spare tube can be placed or the patient awakened. Many of the newer pulse oximeters have been shown to be useful in rodents and lagomorphs (Fig. 14-13). A knowledge of basic physiologic parameters is needed for proper monitoring (Table 14-2).

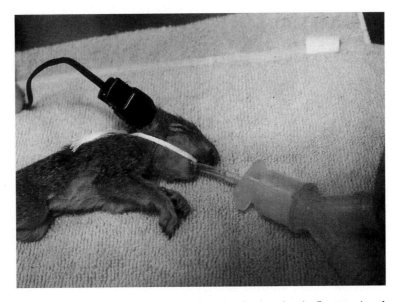

FIGURE 14-13 Squirrel intubated and under anesthesia using isoflurane. A pulse oximeter is being used to aid in the patient's monitoring.

TABLE 14-2 Patient Physiologic Monitoring Data

Species	Respiration/min	Heart rate/min	Body temperature (degrees centigrade)
Chinchilla	40-65	40-100	36.1-37.8
Gerbil	70-120	260-600	38.1-38.4
Guinea pig	42-104	230-380	37.2-39.5
Hamster	35-135	250-500	37.0-38.4
Rabbit	32-60	130-325	38.0-39.6
Rat	70-115	250-450	35.9-37.5

Complete Oral Examination

Once the patient has been stabilized, a more detailed examination of the oral cavity can be undertaken. This will help establish or confirm a diagnosis for an appropriate treatment plan. External palpation, jaw manipulation, and visual and radiographic examination all play a part in an accurate diagnosis of the problem.

Palpation and manipulation

Palpation of the head, face, jaws, and throat area should be carefully performed to locate sites of swellings, discharge, or possible fluid-filled areas, which might indi-

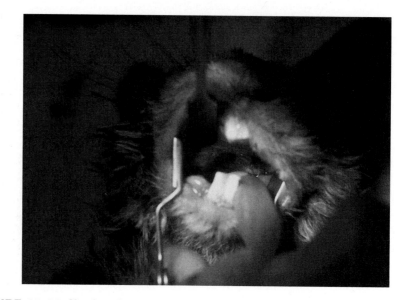

FIGURE 14-14 Cheek and tongue retractors being used to allow proper visualization of the oral cavity and teeth.

cate a pathologic condition. However, small lumps under the ventral mandible beneath the cheek teeth can be a normal anatomic finding in many species.

The jaws should be gently manipulated to examine for resistance to normal occlusal movements. During examination, the practitioner may ask the following questions: Is there reasonable vertical movement, and do the edges of the maxillary and mandibular incisors meet in an appropriate scissors bite? When the mandible is moved from side to side in a horizontal movement, will the jaws remain in a level occlusal plane or is the occlusion forced open on one side and not the other? If uneven movement is noted, the disparity may be caused by an overgrowth of teeth on one side.

Visual examination and aids

The use of a mouth gag, cheek retractors, a tongue retractor, good lighting, and appropriate magnification can greatly enhance the visual examination (Fig. 14-14). When proper soft tissue retraction cannot be attained, visual inspections typically reveal little. While inspecting the teeth, the practitioner should look for hooks, vertical blades of enamel, uneven occlusal beds, and tooth overgrowth. It is common for cheek tooth overgrowth to be on the side of the face opposite that of incisor overgrowth.

Radiographic examination

Radiographs are highly useful diagnostic and monitoring tools for rodents and lagomorphs (Fig. 14-15). The use of intraoral-type dental films is more convenient and can give greater distinction of detail, but standard films can also be used. Several dental film sizes have been found useful for either intraoral or extraoral radiographs. Among these are the sizes No. 0, No. 1, and No. 2 films for actual intraoral

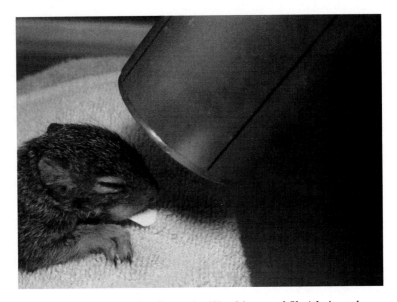

FIGURE 14-15 Intraoral dental radiographs (Size 0 intraoral film) being taken on a young squirrel.

use and the No. 4 size film for extraoral use. Size No. 0-2 can, in some cases, be used intraorally for isolation of the incisor teeth and occasionally the cheek teeth. The No. 4 films used extraorally can be extremely useful diagnostically. They can be used for either a dorsoventral or ventrodorsal and a lateral of the entire head, including dentition and temporomandibular joints. The lateral is commonly the most diagnostically useful of the two views. The lateral view may reveal hooks, overgrowth, uneven occlusal beds, and apical pathology.

Charting

Rodents and lagomorphs should have all detected pathologic conditions charted as thoroughly as possible. The use of charts customized to these species can be helpful but are not absolutely required. (Refer to the index for additional information on charting.)

ORAL TREATMENTS FOR RODENTS AND LAGOMORPHS

Teeth Cleaning

Rodent and lagomorph teeth can be cleaned in a fashion similar to that of most other species (see Chapter 7). However, because of the small oral opening and the risks of fluids running down into the respiratory tract, little or no water spray should be used, particularly if the patient has not been intubated. Therefore hand instruments or mechanical scalers that produce little heat are required; certain sonic and ultrasonic scalers may meet this requirement. The teeth can then be briefly polished. Excess polish and debris should be cleaned from the mouth with cotton swabs.

Floating or Odontoplasty of Teeth

The term *floating* means laying level on a surface or moving gently on a surface. In teeth the term refers to providing a level occlusal surface, which allows for a gentle fluid movement of the teeth. *Odontoplasty* refers to the process of recontouring a tooth surface. Both terms are used almost interchangeably in reference to adjustment of the surface of rabbit or rodent teeth by either abrasion or cutting. Some types of instruments used for adjustment of the teeth include tooth cutters, rasps, files, and various burs and abrasive points.

Tooth cutters

Tooth cutters are available in two types: incisor cutters and molar cutters. They are typically either burs or edge-cutting hand instruments. The edge-cutting hand instruments should generally be used only for cutting spurs and hooks off teeth and **not** for attempting to actually shorten teeth. When used to cut teeth and reduce occlusal height, they are prone to break, crack, or shatter many teeth. Dog toenail clippers should be used carefully if at all.

Incisor cutters

Burs. When cutting incisors, burs on a low- or high-speed handpiece provide not only a smooth, even cut but also the ability to use odontoplasty in reestablishing the chisel-shaped edge, which slopes back and toward the gums from the facial edge. White stone bur points, fluted burs, standard burs, and diamond burs all work well (Fig. 14-16).

Edge-cutting hand instruments. Edge-cutting hand instruments should be used with caution because shattering and crushing effects on the teeth are not unusual. These should be used on incisors only to remove spurs or hooks and not to reduce actual tooth height.

Molar cutters

Burs. When dealing with cheek teeth, most burs and handpieces are difficult to use efficiently and safely because of their rapid cutting and poor visibility in the mouth. However, these instruments can sometimes be used effectively. A low-speed handpiece and a straight handpiece crosscut diamond bur are sometimes useful.

Edge-cutting hand instruments. Because of their visibility and reach, edge-cutting hand instruments are best suited for the removal of spurs and hooks on cheek teeth. However, these instruments are not suitable to cut off actual tooth height; floats are better suited for this process.

Rasps and files

Rasps and files can be used to gradually reduce the height of the cheek teeth while also recontouring them into a reasonable reestablishment of the proper occlusal table angulation (See "Cheek Tooth Occlusal Anatomy") (Fig. 14-17).

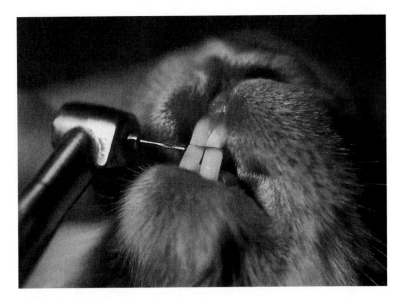

FIGURE 14-16 High-speed dental handpiece with a crosscut bur being used to trim the incisor teeth of a rabbit.

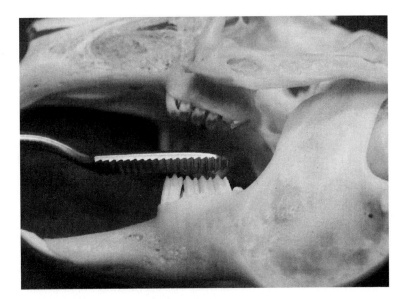

FIGURE 14-17 Demonstration of a float being used on the mandibular cheek teeth of a rabbit skull to level the occlusal surface of the teeth.

Rasps. Because of their construction, rasps usually cut on both the push and pull strokes, which normally results in a more rapid reduction of the tooth surface.

Files. Files cut primarily on the back stroke. This allows for a safer pattern of cutting on the pull stroke from the back of the mouth and normally results in less oral trauma.

Burs and abrasive points
(See "Tooth Cutters.")

Physiologic Floating and Induced Self- or Auto-Floating

A form of physiologic floating of the hypsodont teeth occurs by natural attrition during mastication. This wear normally offsets the continual growth of the teeth, maintaining a balance between the teeth and oral cavity. Induced attrition (induced natural floating) is a technique of manually manipulating the jaws to imitate mastication and force attritional wear. This aids in floating minor spur development and in the finishing process. Induced attrition is usually accomplished while the animal is under anesthesia. It should be performed carefully to prevent additional oral injury and inflammation.

Abscess Treatment

Diseased teeth may develop endodontic, periodontic, and combination periodontic endodontic abscesses. Treatment may involve endodontic procedures, but in general extraction of the diseased tooth is best. The actual abscess may require incision, drainage, and treatment. Most dental-related abscesses are detected by owners, usually on the face or lower jaw. However, some patients are brought in for treatment of other serious secondary problems resulting from inflammation of the diseased teeth.

Endodontic abscesses
Endodontic abscesses frequently result from some form of trauma that has exposed the pulp and resulted in its devitalization or death. Root canals can be performed on these teeth, but long term success is rare. Extraction is in most cases the most prudent approach to treatment. The tooth should be extracted, and the fistulous tract cleaned. The animal should then be placed on antibiotics. If a notable abscess is present, it should also be treated. Treatment of the abscess may include lancing, drainage, flushing, and placement of a drain tube. In some cases the abscess may have caused considerable bone loss in one of the jaws. If this has occurred, a bone replacement material such as Consil® (Nutramax Labs, Baltimore, MD 21236) or HTR® (Bioplant, Inc., South Norwalk, CT 06854) should be considered in an attempt to stimulate new healthy bone growth into the area. The granulation and debris should be removed, the bone replacement material placed in the bony defect, and the lesion closed surgically for first intention healing.

Periodontal abscesses
Abscesses of this nature are typically caused by food or other debris being forced into the periodontal ligament space of a tooth. This results in an abscess along the

gingival or mucosal surface adjacent to the tooth. The abscess should be lanced and cleaned free of any debris, antibiotics should be initiated, and the causative substances should be removed from the diet. Stemmy hays and roughage are often found within these lesions.

Periodontic endodontic abscesses

Periodontic endodontic abscesses are some of the most commonly detected causes of facial or jaw abscesses. These are an extension of periodontic abscesses wherein the infection has traveled down the root of the tooth until it has reached the apex of the tooth. This allows the bacteria access to the endodontic pulp tissues, resulting in an associated endodontic abscess with the periodontic infection or abscess. Treatment is extraction of the diseased tooth, possible placement of a bone replacement material in the alveolus, and initiation of antibiotics.

Extractions

Extractions can be broken down into two categories, depending on whether the tooth is an incisor or cheek tooth. Each type of extraction requires different techniques and equipment. Antibiotics are routinely recommended after most extractions and before the extraction if a serious infection or other preexisting condition warrants the precaution.

Incisor teeth

Incisor teeth can be elevated and extracted in a way similar to the method used for other teeth. However, because of the highly curved clinical root structure and the fragile nature of these teeth and associated bone, use of appropriate technique and equipment is required. Most of the strength of the periodontal ligament holding the tooth in place is found in the gingival third of the ligament and on the mesial surface. This means the primary area to be elevated is the third of the clinical root nearest the gum surface and toward the midline of the mandible. Blunted injection needles sometimes can be quite useful for this purpose. The 18-gauge 1½-inch needle has been used for many years in rabbits. However, the No. 1 and No. 2 Winged Elevators® (Dentalaire, Inc., Fountain Valley, CA 92708) and the Crossley Rabbit Luxator® (Jorgensen Labs, Inc., Loveland, CO 80538) are well designed for this function. Elevation of the tooth is attained by pressing the elevator into the periodontal ligament between the tooth and alveolar bone and gradually rotating it back and forth. This should be done gently because these teeth are fragile, especially when the practitioner is working down the root toward the apex. Once the teeth are loosened, extraction forceps can be used to grasp the tooth and remove it (see Fig. 14-8). The operator should bear in mind that the tooth curves in an arc and the extraction pull must be made in that same circular plane. Once the tooth has been extracted, the empty socket should be cleaned, bone replacement materials placed, and the gums sutured closed with absorbable sutures.

Teeth broken during extraction must be evaluated carefully. These are generally categorized as nondiseased and diseased teeth. Nondiseased teeth are those with no infection or infective pathologic condition, such as a tooth that is extracted because of an atraumatic malocclusion. In these situations the tooth's growth center at the apex may be intact and still active. If this is the case, the tooth will typically regrow in 1 to 4 months, and a second attempt at extraction can be made at that time. Diseased teeth are characterized by infection, pulp exposure, abscess, or traumatic malocclusion. Most are associated with some form of trauma to the tooth or gums. Should one of these teeth be broken, every reasonable attempt should be made to retrieve the broken portion of the tooth because the remaining infected portion usually continues to cause problems. In the effort to remove the remaining segment, Winged Elevators® (Dentalaire, Inc., Fountain Valley, CA 92708), Crossley Rabbit Luxator® (Jorgensen Labs, Inc., Loveland, CO 80538), and a No. 2 Molt surgical elevator (HuFriedy Co., Chicago, IL 60618) are sometimes helpful. If the segment cannot be removed, the open alveolus should be packed with tetracycline powder or gel, such as Heska's Periodontal Therapy Gel (Heska Corp., Fort Collins, CO 80525), and the patient should be prescribed oral antibiotics. If the lost segments continue to cause problems, a surgical approach and curettage will probably be necessary.

Cheek teeth

Extractions of cheek teeth are divided into two categories according to the type of tooth being extracted (brachyodont or aradicular hypsodont). Brachyodont cheek teeth are usually easier to extract than the aradicular hypsodont cheek teeth. These teeth are seen most commonly in rats and mice. The No. 2 Molt surgical elevator (HuFriedy Co., Chicago, IL 60618) and an 18- to 20-gauge injection needle bent at a 90-degree angle work reasonably well as elevators for intraoral extraction of these teeth. In many cases, suturing the extraction site may not be practical. In this case, a hemostatic solution can be applied to the extraction site with a cotton swab to control hemorrhage by pressure and chemical affect, and then several layers of tincture of myrrh and benzoin (Sultan Chem, Englewood, NJ 07631) should be applied as a protective coating. The tincture can be applied with cotton swabs. Each coating should be dried before the next is applied.

Aradicular hypsodont teeth commonly have a more complex and deeper clinical root structure compared with brachyodont teeth. Therefore extractions are usually more difficult. The same basic techniques as previously described for brachyodont teeth can be used, but tooth repelling or even buccotomy may also be required. Tooth repelling is the procedure of making an access hole below the tooth and pressing a small, blunt metal rod against the bottom of the tooth to push it into the oral cavity. In some cases, small, light taps with a small mallet may be required. With many diseased teeth, only light hand pressure is required to accomplish the repelling of the tooth into the mouth. Once accomplished, the access hole should be packed with a bone replacement material and the site sutured closed. The intraoral extraction site may be sutured closed, but if this is too difficult, the previously described treatment, using a hemostatic solution and tincture of myrrh and benzoin, may be used.

Buccotomy is the cutting of the buccal cheek pouch to promote more direct visualization and ability to treat cheek teeth. However, this procedure can leave permanent scars, which some clients may find objectionable. In addition, since many of these species actively use the cheek pouch during eating and may even store food in the pouch, complication of infection and dehiscence of the suture line may occur. Therefore buccotomies should be performed rarely and with some degree of trepidation.

Pulp-Capping

Pulp-capping procedures, performed to maintain tooth vitality, may be required when injury or iatrogenic action causes exposure of the pulp. The site of exposure should be cleaned with sterile saline. The coronal portion of the pulp is removed with a pear-shaped or round bur or a small diamond bur on a high-speed handpiece (partial pulpectomy or pulpotomy). A paper point can be briefly dipped into a Dappen dish of sterile saline. The moistened end is then dipped into a Dappen dish of calcium hydroxide powder. The powder adheres to the paper point, which is then placed into the pulp chamber or canal of the injured tooth until it contacts the pulp. The paper point is then gently tapped against the pulp to displace a small coating of the calcium hydroxide on the pulp. The access is then cleaned, and a restorative, such as a glass ionomer, is placed over the exposure to seal the tooth.

Tooth Fillings

Because of the small size of the teeth generally involved, restoratives that easily bond to enamel and dentine are preferred for fillings. Among these are materials such as the glass ionomers and bonded composites. Due to the required undercuts, cavity preparation, wear resistance, and potential toxic problems, amalgams are seldom used in hypsodont teeth. (For additional information concerning restoratives, consult the index.)

Glass ionomer liners and restoratives are both used for restoration work in rodents and lagomorphs. The lesions should be prepared and the glass ionomer applied according to the manufacturer's recommendations.

Composites, when used with bonding agents, are also well suited for use in rodents and lagomorphs, although they are more technique-sensitive than glass ionomers. Although most types of composite can be used, products that flow easily are often less difficult to apply in the restricted space of these small oral cavities. Reinforced or macro-fill composites should be avoided because their wear pattern might be slower than that of the associated tooth structure.

Because of their metal content (e.g., mercury), amalgams are not recommended for use in aradicular hypsodont teeth. The wear patterns are incompatible, and mercury may be ingested as the material is worn down by attrition.

Drug Treatment

Various antibiotics and other drugs are used in treatment whose dosages must be calculated not only by weight but by species (Table 14-3). **CAUTION:** Some rodents and lagomorphs are sensitive to certain antibiotics; some drugs may even cause death. In rabbits, hamsters, and guinea pigs the potential of fatal colitis caused by the use of antibiotics, especially oral antibiotics, is always present. Chloramphenicol is generally the drug of choice for treatment of this or other enteropathies (see Table 14-3). Therefore antibiotics should be carefully selected and dosages checked before administering. The dosages in Table 14-3 may be useful and have been compiled from various references, but the practitioner must recognize that these dosages are empirical in the dosage and use.

TABLE 14-3 Medications for Pocket Pets

			SPECIES			
	Rabbit	Guinea pig	Chinchilla	Hamster	Gerbils	Rats
Antibiotics						
Amikacin	8-16 mg/kg total dose; once daily to divided tid SQ/IM/IV	10-15 mg/kg total dose; once daily to divided tid SQ/IM/IV	10-15 mg/kg total dose; once daily to divided tid SQ/IM/IV	10-20 mg/kg total dose; once daily to divided tid SQ/IM	10-20 mg/kg total dose; once daily to divided tid SQ/IM	10-20 mg/kg total dose; once daily to divided tid SQ/IM
Chloramphenicol palmitate	50 mg/kg bid PO	50 mg/kg bid PO	50 mg/kg bid PO	50-200 mg/kg tid PO	50-200 mg/kg tid PO	50-200 mg/kg tid PO
Chloramphenicol succinate	30-50 mg/kg bid SQ/IM	30-50 mg/kg bid SQ/IM	30-50 mg/kg bid SQ/IM	30-50 mg/kg SQ/IM	30-50 mg/kg SQ/IM	30-50 mg/kg bid SQ/IM
Chlortetracycline	50 mg/kg bid PO	50 mg/kg bid PO	50 mg/kg PO	20 mg/kg bid SQ/IM		6-10 mg/kg bid SQ/IM
Ciprofloxacin	5-15 mg/kg bid PO	5-15 mg/kg bid PO	5-15 mg/kg bid PO	10 mg/kg bid PO	10 mg/kg bid PO	10 mg/kg bid PO
Doxycycline	2.5 mg/kg bid PO	2.5 mg/kg bid PO	2.5 mg/kg bid PO	2.5 mg/kg bid PO	2.5 mg/kg bid PO	2.5-5 mg/kg bid PO
Enrofloxacin	5-15 mg/kg bid PO/SQ/IM	2.5-10 mg/kg bid PO/SQ/IM	2.5-10 mg/kg bid PO/SQ/IM	2.5-10 mg/kg bid PO/IM		2.5-10 mg/kg bid PO/SQ/IM
Gentamicin	5-8 mg/kg total dose; once daily to divided tid SQ/IM/IV	5-8 mg/kg total dose; once daily to divided tid SQ/IM/IV	5-8 mg/kg total dose; once daily to divided tid SQ/IM/IV	5-8 mg/kg total dose; once daily to divided tid SQ/IM	5-8 mg/kg total dose; once daily to divided tid SQ/IM	5-8 mg/kg total dose; once daily to divided tid SQ/IM/IV
Neomycin	30 mg/kg bid PO	30 mg/kg sid PO	15 mg/kg bid PO	100 mg/kg sid PO	100 mg/kg PO	50 mg/kg sid PO
Penicillin G procaine	20,000 to 60,000 IU/kg					22,000 IU/kg sid SQ/IM

Drug							*Continued*
penicillin and penicillin G procaine	84,000 IU/kg SQ/IM once weekly for 3 weeks						
Sulfadimethoxine	25-50 mg/kg sid PO	25-50 mg/kg sid PO	25-50 mg/kg sid PO	25-50 mg/kg sid PO	25-50 mg/kg sid PO	25-50 mg/kg sid PO	
Sulfamethazine	1-5 mg/ml of drinking water	1-5 mg/ml of drinking water	1-5 mg/ml of drinking water	1-5 mg/ml of drinking water	1-5 mg/ml of drinking water	1-5 mg/ml of drinking water	
Sulfaquinoxaline	1 mg/ml of drinking water	1 mg/ml of drinking water	1 mg/ml of drinking water	1 mg/ml of drinking water	1 mg/ml of drinking water	1 mg/ml of drinking water	
Tetracycline	50 mg/kg bid-tid PO	10-20 mg/kg tid PO	50 mg/kg bid-tid PO	10-20 mg/kg tid PO	10-20 mg/kg tid PO	10-20 mg/kg tid PO	
Trimethoprim/sulfadiazine	30 mg/kg sid-bid SQ	30 mg/kg sid-bid SQ	30 mg/kg sid-bid SQ	30 mg/kg sid SQ	30 mg/kg sid SQ	30 mg/kg sid SQ	
Trimethoprim/sulfamethoxazole	15-30 mg/kg bid PO	15-30 mg/kg bid PO	15-30 mg/kg bid PO	15-30 mg/kg bid PO	15-30 mg/kg bid PO	15-30 mg/kg bid PO	
Tylosin	10 mg/kg bid PO/SQ/IM		2-8 mg/kg bid PO/SQ	10 mg/kg bid PO/SQ/IM	10 mg/kg bid PO/SQ/IM	10 mg/kg bid PO/SQ/IM	

Antiinflammatory

Drug							
Dexamethasone	0.5-2.0 mg/kg bid PO/SQ/IM	0.1-0.6 mg/kg IM		0.1-0.6 mg/kg IM	0.1-0.6 mg/kg IM	0.1-0.6 mg/kg IM	
Prednisone	0.5-2 mg/kg PO	0.5-2 mg/kg PO	0.5-2 mg/kg PO/SQ	0.5-2 mg/kg PO	0.5-2 mg/kg PO	0.5-2 mg/kg PO	

Analgesics

Drug							
Acetaminophen	200-500 mg/kg PO					100-300 mg/kg q4h	
Aspirin	100 mg/kg q4-6h PO	80 mg/kg q4h PO	240 mg/kg PO	240 mg/kg PO	240 mg/kg PO	100 mg/kg q4h PO	

SQ, Subcutaneous; *IM,* intramuscular; *IV,* intravenous; *PO,* per os (by mouth).

TABLE 14-3 Medications for Pocket Pets—cont'd

	Rabbit	Guinea pig	Chinchilla	SPECIES Hamster	Gerbils	Rats
Buprenorphine	0.01-0.1 mg/kg bid-tid SQ/IM/IV	0.05-0.1 mg/kg bid-tid SQ/IM		0.05-1.0 mg/kg bid-tid SQ/IM	0.05-1.0 mg/kg bid-tid SQ/IM	0.05-1.0 mg/kg bid-tid SQ/IM
Butorphanol	0.1-0.5 mg/kg q2-4h SQ/IM/IV	2 mg/kg q2-4h SQ/IM		2 mg/kg q2-4h SQ/IM	2 mg/kg q2-6h SQ/IM	0.5-5 mg/kg q2-6h SQ/IM
Ibuprofen	7.5-20 mg/kg q4h PO	10 mg/kg q4h IM				10-30 mg/kg q4h PO
Other medications						
Acepromazine	1-5 mg/kg IM	0.5-5 mg/kg SQ/IM	0.5-1 mg/kg IM	0.5-5 mg/kg SQ/IM	DO NOT USE	0.5-2.5 mg/kg SQ/IM
Atropine	0.1-0.2 mg/kg IM/SQ	0.05-0.2 mg/kg SQ		0.04-0.2 mg/kg IM	0.04-0.2 mg/kg IM	0.02-0.05 mg/kg IM/SQ
Glycopyrrolate	0.01-0.05 mg/kg IM/SQ	0.01-0.05 mg/kg IM/SQ		0.01-0.05 mg/kg IM/SQ	0.01-0.05 mg/kg IM/SQ	0.01-0.05 mg/kg IM/SQ
Vitamin C		10-30 mg/kg maintenance 50 mg/kg deficiency treatment PO/IM/SQ				

Home-Care Instructions

With regard to small pets, the key point for home care is for the clients to closely observe food and water intake during the first 4 hours after discharge from the clinic. Seriously ill patients may be reluctant to eat and drink after dental procedures. If the patient fails to ingest some food and water within the first 4 hours after treatment, hand feeding with liquid concentrates and water should be instituted until normal intake resumes. Prolonged inappetence is generally an indication of a more severe secondary problem, which may require administration of fluids, antibiotics, antiinflammatories, and additional supportive care and treatments, as well as patient reassessment.

Worksheet

STUDENT NAME: _____

1. Lagomorphs have _____ _____ teeth that continually grow throughout the animal's life, whereas rodents may have _____ and _____ teeth.

2. Rodents and lagomorphs have a heterodont form of dentition and have _____, _____, and _____, but no _____ teeth.

3. The periodontal ligament of hypsodont teeth has an _____, which allows for continued growth and eruption of the teeth.

4. Malocclusions are generally grouped in two categories: _____ or _____.

5. _____ malocclusions are normally associated with some form of trauma to the teeth that has resulted in broken teeth and the overgrowth of their opposing dentition.

6. When the tongue is pinned to the roof of the mouth by tooth overgrowth, the patient is described as being _____.

7. When food accumulates and hardens in the oral pouches, the condition is called _____.

8. _____ is the discrepancy of widths of the upper and lower jaws.

9. The classic bright yellow/orange color on the facial surfaces of the incisor teeth is actually the _____ _____.

10. Food and water should be restricted for how long before surgery on rodents and lagomorphs? _____.

REFERENCES

Wiggs RB, Lobprise HB: Dental and oral disease in rodents and lagomorphs. In *Veterinary dentistry principles and practice,* Philadelphia, 1997, Lippincott-Raven.

Wiggs RB, Lobprise HB: Oral anatomy and physiology of pet rodents and lagomorphs. In Penman S, Crossley DA, editors: *Manual of small animal dentistry,* Gloucestershire, UK, 1995, British Small Animal Association.

Wiggs RB, Lobprise HB: Oral diagnosis in pet rodents and lagomorphs. In Penman S, Crossley DA, editors: *Manual of small animal dentistry,* Gloucestershire, UK, 1992, British Small Animal Association.

Wiggs RB, Lobprise HB: Prevention and treatment of dental problems in rodents and lagomorphs. In Penman S, Crossley DA, editors: *Manual of small animal dentistry,* Gloucestershire, UK, 1992, British Small Animal Association.

Lobprise HB, Wiggs RB: Dental and oral disease in lagomorphs, *J Vet Dent* 8(2):11, 1991.

Wiggs RB, Lobprise HB: Dental and oral disease in rodents, *J Vet Dent* 7(3):6, 1990.

Hillyer EV, Quesenberry KE: *Ferrets, rabbits and rodents: clinical medicine and surgery,* Philadelphia, 1997, WB Saunders.

Allen DG, Pringle JK, Smith DA: *Handbook of veterinary drugs,* ed 2, Philadelphia, 1998, Lippincott-Raven.

Muir WW and others: *Handbook of veterinary anesthesia,* ed 2, St Louis, 1995, Mosby.

15

Marketing Veterinary Dentistry

Marketing is a system of activities designed to identify and satisfy consumer needs and desires. During the patient examination the veterinarian must determine the patient's medical needs and then inform the clients in such a manner that they want the services. The first step in effectively marketing a product or service is to determine the patient's needs. In veterinary medicine, practitioners must first educate themselves and become familiar with all aspects of the anticipated service. However, despite what many practitioners assume, marketing is more than merely presenting this information to the client. In reality, marketing begins with developing your product through education.

Another way to look at marketing is that it is really "doctoring." It entails examining the patient, advising the client on the needs of the patient, and advising the client on the capability of the practice to deliver the recommended services. A variety of methods reinforce the importance of veterinary dentistry in maintaining overall health.

MARKETING STRATEGIES

Practice Brochures

The investment of time, effort, and money in the creation of a practice brochure can be extremely rewarding. The practice brochure should cover all aspects of service, including, of course, dental procedures. The brochure may provide information on practice policies, equipment, and commonly performed procedures; with the addition of illustrations, it can also be a pictorial guide to the practice.

Smile Book

A "smile book" is a pictorial description of procedures performed in the practice. One effective strategy is to include "before and after" photographs of dental procedures. This type of visual aid can be used to educate the client with regard to expected outcomes. It also can be used to describe the various steps of a recommended procedure or alternative procedure.

Posters and Transparencies

A variety of posters and transparencies are available that graphically illustrate dental disease (Figs. 15-1 and 15-2). Some posters can be framed and hung in the reception area or exam room. Others can be backlit in the exam room on x-ray view boxes.

Newsletters

The practice newsletter should include a section on dentistry. Potential topics include the following: cause of periodontal disease, treatment techniques for the prevention and treatment of periodontal disease, fractured teeth, dietary considerations in dentistry, veterinary dental orthodontics, cervical line lesions, and dental home-care products. Clip art, which is available from several commercial sources, can be used to enliven the textual content.

Messages on Hold

Rather than listening to music (or, worse yet, silence) while they are on hold, clients can hear informative messages about veterinary medicine and veterinary dentistry. Subjects may include the need to take care of teeth, periodontal disease, fractured teeth, home care, and other important information.

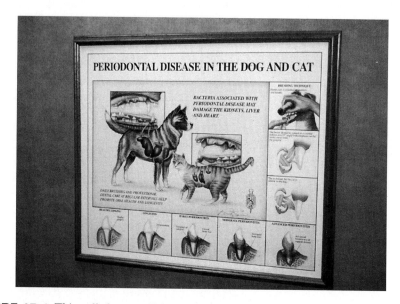

FIGURE 15-1 This wall chart, available though Virbac, describes possible systemic disease caused by periodontal disease, stages of periodontal disease, and proper tooth-brushing techniques.

Handouts

Handouts give the client additional information on the procedure or procedures that must be performed. Several pharmaceutical companies distribute helpful handouts and transparencies that may mention the company's products on the back page but focus primarily on delivering objective information (see Fig. 15-2). Handouts are also available for purchase through commercial companies.

The practice can also customize and print original handouts. This allows customization of the handout to inform the client of the need for the procedure. Handouts can be general, covering all branches of veterinary dentistry, or specific, dealing only with the procedure recommended for the particular patient. Handouts on periodontal disease should cover the need for prevention through the complete prophy. Handouts on endodontic disease should discuss the reasons for performing root canals and the consequence of no treatment. The preoperative handout can be in the form of a dental estimate that discusses fees, expected outcomes, and possible complications associated with the individual patient's disease process.

Some practices have computer systems that can generate handouts on demand. For example, after a patient with Stage 1 disease undergoes a prophy, a handout describing the stage of the disease, treatment, and home care can be linked to the computerized record. This handout would be different for the patient with Stage 4 periodontal disease undergoing periodontal therapy.

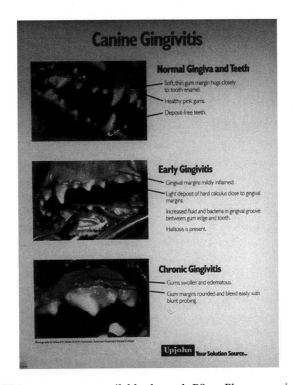

FIGURE 15-2 This transparency, available through Pfizer Pharmaceuticals, demonstrates various aspects of periodontal disease.

Estimate and Consent Forms

Although designed primarily for legal reasons, estimate and consent forms are valuable marketing tools. An estimate is an effective way to present the treatment plan before the procedure is performed. Unfortunately, many veterinarians determine their fees after they have already performed the procedure; usually, they decide that they are charging too much and subtract charges where they can. To be fair to the practice and client, the best method is to document all necessary costs beforehand. Developing a treatment plan and estimate is an excellent way to promote discussion of the patient's needs and the client's wishes.

Of course, during the course of one procedure, practitioners often discover a need for another. One method to handle this is to give the client three choices on the standard estimate/surgical release/drop off form. These choices may be presented as follows:
1. Do anything the doctor feels necessary.
2. Call first; if I cannot be reached, do what is necessary.
3. Do nothing if you cannot contact me.

These three questions eliminate the frustration of trying to contact a client who is difficult to reach while the patient is under anesthesia.

Recall System

Recall cards are a valuable method of reminding the client to return for repeat visits. Recall reminders should be customized according to the patient's needs. Clients with generally healthy pets and pets with gingivitis should be reminded to come in for annual visits. Patients with established periodontal disease should be seen every 3 to 6 months, and patients with advanced periodontal disease should be seen every 3 months.

Dental Models

Plastic dental models are available for use in client education (Fig. 15-3). This education should focus on the patient's condition and recommended procedures for treatment. Three companies currently distribute plastic dental models of the canine and feline oral anatomy and disease conditions. Butler Company (800-344-2246) and Henry Schein Company (800-872-4346) market models with excellent representations of dental abnormalities and pathology. Dr. Shipp's Laboratories (800-442-0107) offer models with plastic teeth embedded in clear plastic. All three varieties are excellent for demonstrating root structure.

Special Events

Many practices sponsor special events to draw attention to dental health. These are an excellent way to increase awareness of this important aspect of veterinary medicine, and the entire staff can become involved. Participation in National Pet Dental Health Month (currently in February) allows the practice to use professional resources for advertising and other materials. In "Pet Dental Checks" veterinarians

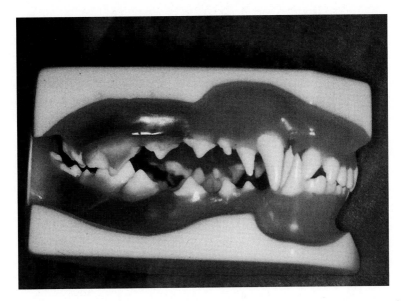

FIGURE 15-3 Dental models can be used to show dental disease, demonstrate techniques of tooth-brushing, and reinforce the need for dental care.

perform exams (focusing on the oral cavity) on large numbers of patients. Clients receive report cards after participating. "The Great Brush Off" is a contest demonstrating tooth-brushing techniques and dog obedience. A "Dog Walk" can be a community "fun run" or walk. These can be tied into "Pet Dental Checks." Veterinarians and staff can also host booths at health fairs intended for human health. These opportunities vary from area to area and practice to practice.

MARKETING IN THE EXAM ROOM

A dental exam should be conducted when the patient is 7 to 8 months of age to evaluate the occlusion and ensure that all primary teeth have exfoliated. At this time, further education may be provided to the client. Suggested topics include the recognition of dental disease, the importance of brushing and other home-care techniques, breed predilection for dental disease, and the need for regular professional teeth cleaning. If the patient is going under general anesthesia for spaying or neutering, the teeth can be scaled (or even just polished) at that time. Dental exams should be included with the annual physical and may correspond with routine teeth-cleaning appointments. The key is to prevent disease, not let it start and then attempt to treat it. Dental exams for older patients should be performed as appropriate; some require dental procedures every 3 months, and others yearly. Patients with periodontal disease should be rechecked every 1 to 2 weeks until the condition is under control. The patient should be recalled every 3 months to make sure that oral health is being maintained. Patients with cervical line lesions should be checked 3 months after treatment to make sure the restoration is still in place. Patients that have had endodontic procedures (pulp-capping or root canal therapy) should be rechecked and radiographed under general anesthesia 6 months after the procedure.

Every patient that comes through the practice door has a mouth, and in these mouths are many problems that must be solved. Each problem may be viewed as a marketing opportunity and a way to provide better service to the patient.

Worksheet

STUDENT NAME: _____

1. Traditionally, marketing is defined as a system of activities to

   _____ and _____ consumer

   _____ and _____.

2. Realistically, however, marketing is also _____.

3. A "_____ _____" is a pictorial

   description of procedures performed in the practice.

4. A variety of _____ are available that graphically

   illustrate dental disease.

5. _____ give the client more information on the

   procedure or procedures that need to be performed.

6. Computerized _____ may link the information

   presented to the individual patient's dental disease.

7. _____ _____ are a valuable method of

   reminding the client to return for repeat visits.

8. _____ (month) is National Pet Dental Health Month.

9. A dental exam should be conducted when the patient is 7 to 8

   months of age to evaluate the _____.

10. Each problem that needs to be solved can be viewed as a

    marketing opportunity and a way to provide _____

    _____ to the patient.

16

Commonly Asked Questions

Topic	Question	Answer
Anesthesia—monitors	What type of monitors are used for anesthesia?	(Check with the doctor for information about specific types of monitors used in the hospital.) The patient is monitored with a pulse oximeter, which measures the amount of oxygen in the blood; a blood-pressure monitor, an electrocardiogram, and an end-tidal CO_2 monitor. That way, the staff is always aware of the patient's condition during anesthesia.
Anesthesia—risk	What is the risk of anesthesia? (Or a variation of the same question, "Is my pet too old for anesthesia?")	Generally, anesthesia poses much less of a risk than untreated periodontal disease. The actual risk needs to be evaluated by the doctor because each patient is different. Blood profiles, chest x-rays, and other tests may be taken before the procedure to fully evaluate the risk.
Bad breath	Why does my dog have such bad breath, and why does it keep getting worse?	Although other causes are possible, bad breath is usually caused by periodontal disease. An oral examination is necessary for proper evaluation.
Discolored tooth	My pet's tooth is purple; what's wrong?	A purple tooth is usually caused by trauma. Most of the time, these teeth are dying and require root canal therapy. These teeth should be examined and treated. Dental radiographs may also be necessary.
Dropping food	My cat picks up his food and drops it; sometimes his mouth opens and closes rapidly when this happens. Why?	Dropping food may be a sign of tooth pain caused by a condition similar to tooth decay. This cat should be examined; dental radiographs may also be necessary.
Drooling	Why does my pet drool?	Excessive drooling may be secondary to dental disease; examination is necessary.

Continued

Topic	Question	Answer
Extractions— reasons	Why must my pet's teeth be pulled?	Teeth must be extracted because of severe periodontal disease, fractures, resorptive lesions, malalignment, and other problems that cause discomfort or difficulty in chewing.
Fractured tooth	My pet's tooth is fractured. What should I do?	Only two choices for treatment are practical. The veterinarian may extract the tooth or perform root canal therapy. Leaving it alone will result in infection of the pulp (probably already present), which can cause pain and other medical problems. Even if the pet is eating and acting normal, the fracture should be addressed.
Fees— "sticker shock"	We just moved here, and my dog needs to have her teeth cleaned under general anesthesia. Why is it so expensive?	Veterinary fees are based on expenses. The least expensive care is not necessarily the best bargain. To cut fees, the veterinarian may have to eliminate something (the best anesthesia, training, anesthesia monitoring equipment, and other dental equipment).
Loose teeth	My pet's teeth are loose; what should I do?	Loose teeth are caused by fractures, periodontal disease, cancer, and many other problems. An examination and possibly dental radiographs are recommended.
Retained primary teeth	My pet has both baby and adult teeth in place. What should I do?	This is a common problem, particularly in small breeds. The baby teeth must be surgically removed to allow sufficient room for the adult teeth.
Scaling teeth	Can I scale my pet's teeth at home?	There is no way for the client to scale the pet's teeth at home because it must be done when the pet is under anesthesia. After the initial scaling by the veterinarian, the client can help maintain the pet's oral health by daily tooth brushing.
Swollen face	My dog has a swelling below his eye that seems to come and go. What is wrong?	The patient probably has a broken upper premolar tooth that requires treatment. Broken premolars are usually caused by eating cow hooves, bones, or other hard objects.
Teeth—Number	How many teeth does my cat have?	30
Teeth—Number	How many teeth does my dog have?	42
Toothbrushing— how often?	How often should I brush my pet's teeth?	For best results, teeth should be brushed daily. (For a more thorough explanation, see Chapter 8.)

Continued

Topic	Question	Answer
Toothbrushing—does not help	My dog has dirty teeth. I have tried cleaning them myself with canine toothpaste and a brush, but it doesn't seem to help much. I do not want my pet to undergo general anesthesia. Is there anything else I can do? His gums bleed sometimes.	Teeth must be cleaned to remove calculus; to do this thoroughly and completely, anesthesia is necessary. Then, the client can brush the patient's teeth twice daily to maintain good oral health.
Tooth wear	My 10-year-old dog is slowly losing her front bottom teeth. They seem to be sensitive, and it looks as though she has ground her teeth down to nubs. Will they fall out? What can I do for her?	Teeth can wear down because of friction against other teeth. Wear is also caused by chewing foreign objects and even skin and hair. The best thing to do is to schedule an exam. Treatment ranges from extraction to root canal therapy.

Dental Equipment Inventory

HOSPITAL INVENTORY

The following table lists minimal equipment requirements that, in the author's opinion, are necessary to perform the treatments indicated. Many alternatives to the items mentioned here exist; this list is meant to be a starting point only!

Basic

Hospitals provide basic prophy and exodontic services only. (Dental radiology services are recommended for the proper performance of exodontics.)

Item	Suggested	Number	Location
Safety glasses or face shield	t		
Respirator mask	t/day		
Exam gloves	*		
Ultrasonic scaler	One		
#3 Ultrasonic insert	*		
#10 Ultrasonic insert	*		
Periodontal tip insert	*		
Sickle scaler (H6/7, N6/7, SH6/7 or Cislak P-12)	*		
Curette (Barnhardt 5/6 or Cislak P-10)	*		
Periodontal probe/explorer	*		
Compressed air system	One		
Slow-speed handpiece or electric motor handpiece	Two		

Continued

Item	Suggested	Number	Location
Prophy angle	*		
Prophy cups	Package		
Prophy paste—coarse	Package or jar		
Prophy paste—fine	Package or jar		
Disclosing solution	One bottle		
Prophy angle lubricant	One bottle		
High-speed handpiece spray	One can		
Arkansas sharpening stone	One		
Arkansas conical sharpening stone	One		
High-speed handpiece	Two		
701 L Burs	One package		
301ss Elevator	×		
301s or Cislak EX-5	×		
301s (modified) or Cislak EX-5H	Two		
301 or Cislak EX 4	×		
303 or Cislak EX-3	×		
Root tip picks—Heibrink, HB10/11, Cislak 14 or Miltex 76	×		
Feline extraction forceps	×		
Periosteal elevator—Molt #9	Two		
Thumb forceps	×		
Mayo-Hegar needle holder	×		
4-0 Dexon, Maxon, or Vicryl suture	Package		
Consil®	Box		

Intermediate

Hospital provides basic prophy services, dental radiography, and the treatment of periodontal disease.

Items in the basic list, plus the following:

Item	Suggested	Number	Location
Dental x-ray machine	One		
Chairside darkroom	One		
X-ray developing solution	Bottle		
X-ray fixing solution	Bottle		
X-ray developing clips	Six		
Size 0, DF 57 x-ray film	Box		
Size 2, DF 58 x-ray film	Box		
Size 4, DF 50 x-ray film	Box		
X-ray film mounts	Box		
HESKA Therapeutic	Box		
No. 3 (or similar) scalpel handle	×		
Small tissue scissors (LaGrange)	One		
Sterile saline solution	Bottle		
#15c Blades	Box		

Advanced

Hospital provides all veterinary dental services.

Items in the Basic and Intermediate plus:

Item	Suggested	Number	Location
Light curing gun	One		
Assorted burs: tapered crosscut fissure burs, 701L; round burs, #2, #4; pear-shaped burs, #330	Minimum five each type		
31-mm K-files: 06, 08, 10, 15, 20, 25, 30, 35, 40, 45, 50, 55, 60, 70, 80, 90, 100	Minimum six each type		
45-mm K-files: 06, 08, 10, 15, 20, 25, 30, 35, 40, 45, 50, 55, 60, 70, 80, 90, 100	Minimum six each type		
60-mm Hedström files: 30, 35, 40, 45, 50, 55, 60, 70, 80	Minimum six each type		
Endodontic stops	One per file (placed on file before use)		
Endodontic irrigation needles, 27 gauge	Box		
Barbed broaches—assorted sizes	Minimum two each		
Endodontic rings	One		
Endodontic sponges	Bag		
RC-Prep	Syringe		
Canal irrigant: sodium hypochlorite, chlorhexidine	Sock bottle plus Luer lock syringe		
Paper absorbent points: similar size to files	Packages		
Root canal sealer: ZOE or advanced sealers	One box		
Mixing pad	One pad		
Mixing spatula	One		
Endodontic point forceps: cotton or college pliers	One		

Continued

Item	Suggested	Number	Location
#30 Plugger and spreader	One		
#50 Plugger and spreader	One		
#65 Plugger and spreader	One		
#90 Plugger and spreader	One		
Light cure restorative materials	One		
Finishing disks, points, or stones	Box		
Impression trays	One set		
Impression material: alginate	Jar		
Laboratory stone	Box		
Dental lab vibrator	One		
Bite registration material	Box		
Orthodontic cement	Box		
Orthodontic buttons	Box		
Howe pliers	One		
Flour pumice	Jar		
Power cord—assorted sizes	Reel		
Band-removing forceps			

* = Maximum number of prophy/periodontal therapy/day × 1 (this allows sterilization for each patient).
† = One per technician.
× = Maximum number of extractions/day × 1 (this allows sterilization for each patient).

Bibliography

Bellows J: *The practice of veterinary dentistry: a team effort,* Ames, Iowa, 1999, Iowa State University Press.

Bojrab MJ, Tholen M: *Small animal medicine and surgery,* Philadelphia, 1989, Lea & Febiger.

Eisenmenger E, Zetner K: *Veterinary dentistry,* Philadelphia, 1985, Lea & Febiger.

Emily P, Penman S: *Handbook of small animal dentistry,* Oxford, 1990, Pergamon Press.

Harvey CE, Emily P: *Small animal dentistry,* ed 2, St Louis, Mosby (in press).

Harvey CE: *Veterinary dentistry,* Philadelphia, 1985, WB Saunders.

Holmstrom SE, Frost P, Gammon RG: *Veterinary dental techniques for the small animal practitioner,* Philadelphia, 1992, WB Saunders.

Holmstrom SE, Frost P, Eisner ER: *Veterinary dental techniques for the small animal practitioner,* Philadelphia, 1998, WB Saunders.

Holmstrom SE, guest editor: *The veterinary clinics of North America small animal practice, canine dentistry,* Philadelphia, 1998, WB Saunders.

Mulligan TW, Aller MS, Williams CA: *Atlas of canine and feline dental radiography,* Trenton, N.J., 1998, Veterinary Learning Systems.

Page RC, Schroeder HE: *Periodontitis in man and other animals,* New York, 1982, Karger.

Shipp AD, Fahrenkrug P: *Practitioners' guide to veterinary dentistry,* Beverly Hills, Calif, 1992, Dr. Shipp's Labs Publishing.

Tholen MA: *Concepts in veterinary dentistry,* Edwardsville, Kan, 1983, Veterinary Medicine Publishing.

Verstraete FJM, editor: *Self-assessment color review of veterinary dentistry,* Ames, Iowa, 1999, Iowa State University Press.

Wiggs RB, Lobprise HB: *Veterinary dentistry principles and practice,* Philadelphia, 1997, Lippincott-Raven.

Wilkins EM: *Clinical practice of the dental hygienist,* Baltimore, 1994, Williams & Wilkins.

Additional Recommended Reading

Journal of Veterinary Dentistry, obtained by membership in the American Veterinary Dental Society: (800) 332-AVDS (2837).

Index